Jesuit Health Sciences & the Promotion of Justice

An Invitation to a Discussion

In Memory of David C. Thomasma (1939-2002)

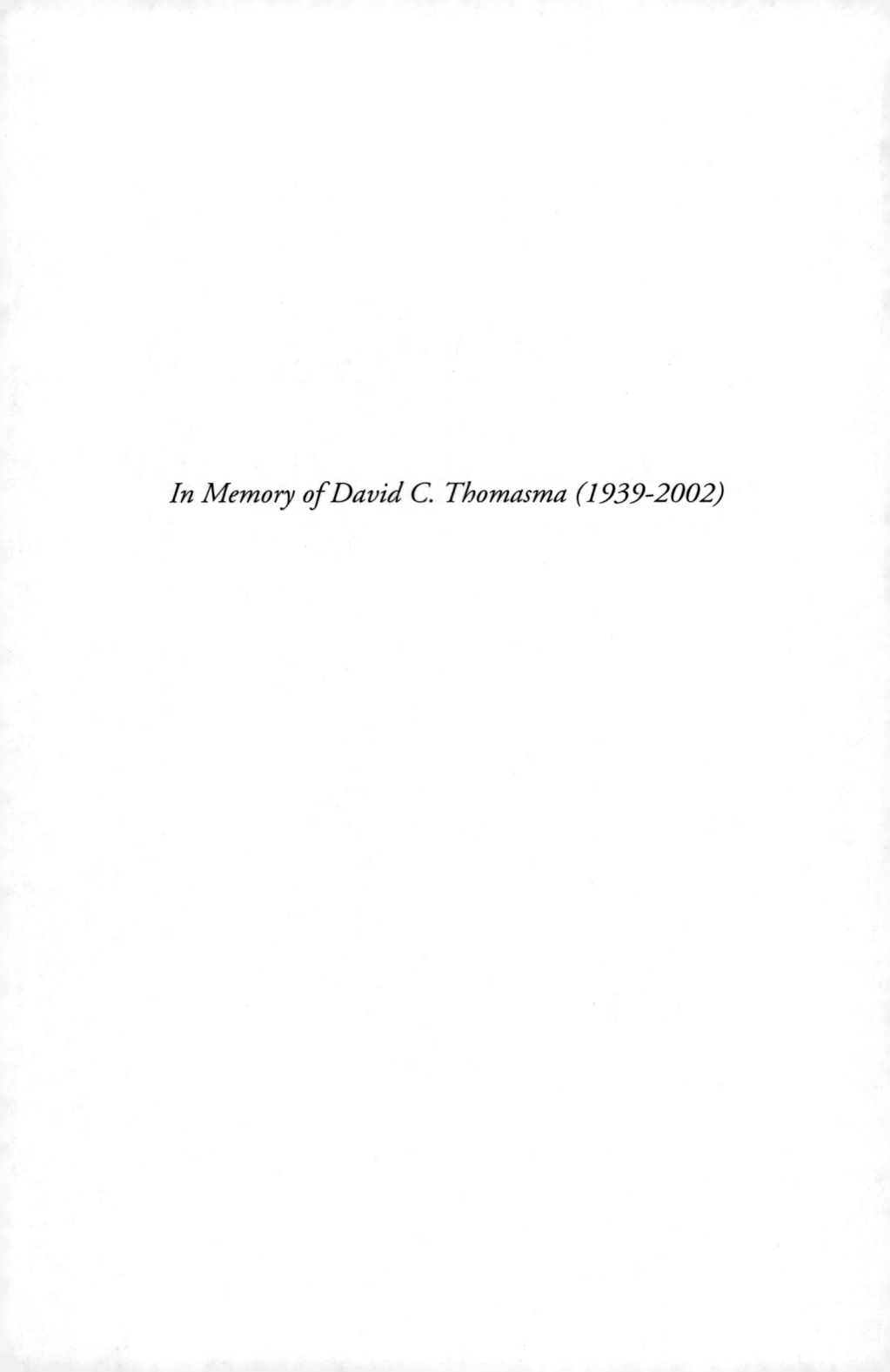

Jesuit Health Sciences & the Promotion of Justice
An Invitation to a Discussion

Jos V.M. Welie
&
Judith Lee Kissell

Editors

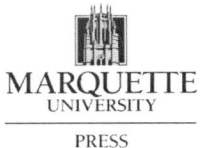

Marquette Studies in Theology
No. 42
Andrew Tallon, Series Editor

Library of Congress Cataloging-in-Publication Data

Jesuit health sciences and the promotion of justice : an invitation to a discussion / Jos V.M. Welie & Judith Lee Kissell, editors.
  p. ; cm. — (Marquette studies in theology ; #42)
Includes bibliographical references and index.
ISBN 0-87462-694-3 (pbk. : alk. paper)
1. Medical sciences—Study and teaching. 2. Medical ethics. 3. Jesuits—Education. 4. Christianity and justice—Catholic Church. 5. Medicine—Religious aspects—Catholic Church. 6. Catholic Church—Doctrines.
[DNLM: 1. Education, Medical. 2. Religion and Medicine. 3. Christianity. W 18 J58 2004] I. Welie, Jos V. M. II. Kissell, Judith Lee. III. Series.
R737.J47 2004
610'.71'1--dc22
                              2004018375

© 2004
Marquette University Press
Milwaukee, Wisconsin USA
All rights reserved.
Second Printing, 2007
Third Printing, 2008

Cover photo by Don Doll, S.J.

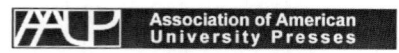

MARQUETTE UNIVERSITY PRESS
MILWAUKEE

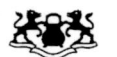

The Association of Jesuit University Presses

Table of Contents

1. *Jos V.M. Welie & Judith Lee Kissell*
   A Matter of Identity: The Role of Jesuit Health Sciences Centers toward the Promotion of Justice. 9

PART I: THE QUEST FOR IDENTITY

2. *Kirk Peck*
   A Historical Perspective on Jesuit Higher Education and a Personal Reflection of a Physical Therapy Professor 19
   I. Living the Jesuit Mission: A Personal Reflection 19
   II. A Short History of the Mission Debate in Catholic Higher Education 23
   III. The Vatican Response to Catholic Identity 26
   IV. Early Jesuit Education 30
   V. Ignatian Spirituality, the *Spiritual Exercises*, and Jesuit Education ... 31
   VI. Towards a "Well-ordered" Plan: *The Ratio Studiorum* 33
   VII. Contemporary Ignatian Pedagogy 35
   VIII. Living the Jesuit Mission: Creighton University 40
   IX. Living the Jesuit Mission: A Personal Reflection Continued 41

3. *Peter-Hans Kolvenbach, SJ*
   The Service of Faith and the Promotion of Justice in American Jesuit Higher Education 49
   I. Introduction 49
   II. The Jesuit Commitment to Faith and Justice—New in 1975 50
      A. The Service of Faith 52
      B. The Promotion of Justice 53
      C. The Ministry of Education 55
   III. A "Composition" of Our Time and Place 57
   IV. American Jesuit Higher Education for Faith and Justice 59
      A. Formation and Learning 59
      B. Research and Teaching 61
      C. Our Way of Proceeding 63
   V. In Conclusion—an Agenda 64

4. *Thomas Massaro, SJ*
   A Preferential Option for the Poor: Historical and Theological Foundations 69

I. Introduction 69
II. The Turn toward Justice 70
III. The Poor in the Scriptures 72
IV. A Case Study in Institutionalizing an Option for the Poor:
    The Jesuits of Latin America 82
V. Paying the Price 85
VI. The Task Ahead: Applying the Lessons of this Case Study to
    US Health Care and Health Sciences Systems 89

PART II: JUSTICE AS THE HALLMARK OF JESUIT HEALTH SCIENCES EDUCATION

5. *Walter Burghardt, SJ*
   Biblical Justice and "The Cry of the Poor": Jesuit Medicine and the
   Third Millennium 95
   I. Signs of the Times 96
      A. Connection between Social Ills and Illness 97
      B. Cries to the Poor 97
      C. Resurgence of Rugged Individualism 101
   II. Jesuit Medicine for a Third Millennium 102
      A. Biblical Justice 103
      B. Relationship with a Person 104
      C. Preferential Option for Community 106

6. *Jos VM Welie*
   "For Whom and For What?" Education and Research in the
   Medical and Dental Sciences 111
   I. Introduction 111
   II. Education for Justice in the Health Sciences 116
   III. The Historical Origins of Jesuit Health Sciences 122
   IV. Contemporary Health Sciences Education for Justice ..124
   V. Concluding Reflections 127

7. *William E. Stempsey, SJ*
   Forming Physicians for the Poor: The Role of Medical and
   Premedical Education 131
   I. Introduction 131
   II. The Problem: Changing Attitudes 133
   III. Premedical Education and Medical School Admissions 140
   IV. Teaching Care for the Poor in Medical School 143
   V. Conclusion 149

Contents

PART III: EXAMPLES AT WORK

8. *Rachel Bognet*
A Service Mission to Haiti Sponsored by the
Medical Alumni Council 155
  I. A Project developed by Scranton's Medical Alumni 155
  II. The Experience of an Undergraduate Pre-Med Student 156

9. *Frank Bernt & Peter Clark, SJ*
An Interdisciplinary, International Approach to Justice in Health 161
  I. Justice and the Pre-Med Undergraduate Curriculum 161
  II. A New Course: Just Health Care in Developing Nations 162
  III. Food for Thought 166

10. *Miriam Schulman*
Experiencing Ethics: Undergraduate Community-Based Learning in a
Local Acute Care Hospital 169

11. *Judith Lee Kissell*
Teaching Medical Students about Vulnerable Patients:
  A Course Example 175
  I. Introduction 175
  II. The Nuts and Bolts 176
  III. Structure and Schedule 178
  IV. Written Assignments 182
  V. Conclusion 183

12. *Frank Ayers*
Creighton's Institute for Latin American Concern: A Unique Opportunity
  to Provide Dental Care to an Underserved Population 185
  I. The History of the ILAC Program 186
  II. The Current ILAC Summer Program 188

13. *Robin Y. Wood*
Bringing Preventive Health Care to a Forgotten Population:
  A Nursing Research Project about Breast Cancer Screening among
  Older Black and White Women 193
  I. Mission and Research 193
  II. Background Information 194

8 *Jesuit Health Sciences & the Promotion of Justice*

III. The Study 195
IV. The Results 197
V. Conclusions 198

14. *Rosanna DeMarco & Anne Norris*
Women's Voices Women's Lives:
A Web-Based HIV Prevention Film Project 203
I. The Background 203
II. The Web-Based Intervention Project 205

15. *Marylou Yam*
Survivors of Intimate Partner Abuse: A Nursing Research Project 211
I. Justice and Nursing Research 211
II. The Proposed Study: An Intervention to Increase Self-Efficacy and Health Promotion Behaviors and Decrease Depression among Women Who Have Experienced Intimate Partner Abuse 212

16. *Julie Sanford*
Researching the Health Status of the Rural Caregiver 219

PART IV: ADMINISTRATIVE COMMENTARIES

17. *Fortunato Cristobal*
Toward Unity for Health in Medical Education:
A Case from the Philippines 227
I. Health in our Region 227
II. Planning a Medical School for Unity of Health and Development . 227
III. The Beginnings—Vision and Mission 228

18. *André Piront, SJ*
Forming Future Physicians: A Report from Belgium 231

19. *F. Daniel Davis*
The Jesuit Medical School and its Leadership Role in
Healing Medical Education 235

PART V: APPENDICES

20. Documents on Jesuit Health Care and Health Sciences Education . 243
21. Contributors 247
22. Index 253

1. Jos V.M. Welie & Judith Lee Kissell

A Matter of Identity: The Role of Jesuit Health Sciences Centers toward the Promotion of Justice

> The preferential option for the poor is not simply an "option" for Christians. It is an obligation to choose to care for the poor to a greater extent than that found in secular society
>
> Pellegrino & Thomasma
> *Helping and Healing*

Ever since the founding of the Society of Jesus by the Basque soldier-convert Ignatius of Loyola in the mid-15th century, the Society has been engaged in social activism, caring for the poor and marginalized, striving to improve their lot through practical care, education and political engagement. A worldwide missionary network as had never existed before was established in a mere century. All of this came to an abrupt end when in the late 18th century, the civil authorities of Spain and France began to expel the Jesuits, culminating in the abolishment of the Society by Pope Clement XIV in 1773. The network collapsed and virtually all of the schools and other missionary institutions were closed. Four decades later, Pope Pius VII realized the error of his predecessor and in 1814 reestablished the Society. But the damage was done; the fire had gone. The Society slowly reemerged but it would be a much more reserved Society, careful not to step on powerful toes.

In 1965 yet another Basque was elected to become the 28th Superior General of the Society. A former medical student, eye witness of the horrors of Hiroshima, Father Arrupe would once again change the image of the Society. In his address to the attendees of the International Congress of Jesuit Alumni in Valencia, Spain, on July 31, 1973, Arrupe asked:

> Have we Jesuits educated our alumni for justice? We will have to answer, in all sincerity, that we have not. This means that, in the future, we must make sure that the education imparted in Jesuit schools will be equal to the demands of justice in the world.... What kind of person is needed today by the world? My shorthand is "men and women for others".... Only by being a man or woman for others does a person become fully human. Only in this way can we live in the Spirit of Jesus Christ, who gave of himself for the salvation of the world, who was, above all others, a man-for-others.

In 1975 the Jesuits delegated to the Society's 32nd General Congregation affirmed that the Society's mission was "the service of faith, of which the promotion of justice is an absolute requirement" *(Decrees of the 31st and 32nd General Congregations of the Society of Jesus*, 1977, p. 411). This mission became once again the hallmark of the Society—one that should pervade all of its missions, including higher education. Joseph Daoust, SJ, has pointed out that the 34th General Congregation discerned these ways in which Jesuit institutions can promote justice: "(1) direct[ing] service and accompaniment of the poor; (2) developing awareness of the demands of justice and the social responsibility to achieve it; (3) participating in social mobilization for the creation of a more just social order." He goes on to argue that neither the first nor the third is "at the heart of what the educational enterprise is about; soup kitchens and political mobilization campaigns are organized around these ways of 'doing' justice. But the second level, developing social consciousness and conscience, or "conscientization," as the Latin Americans call it, is of the essence of Jesuit education" (Daoust, 1999).

In the late 1990s, the presidents from three of America's Jesuit universities (Maureen Fay of University of Detroit Mercy, Bill Leahy of Boston College and Paul Locatelli of Santa Clara), immediately followed by the other 25 presidents, initiated a process of self-study. They recalled the question Father Arrupe had raised 25 years earlier: Are the Jesuit colleges and universities educating for justice? Regional

A Matter of Identity

conferences were then held in 1999 followed by a national meeting at Santa Clara University in 2000 (see elsewhere in this volume for the complete text of his presentation). There Father Arrupe's successor, Peter-Hans Kolvenbach, addressed the gathered presidents and university representatives. Where Arrupe had focused on education, Kolvenbach expanded the agenda. The service of faith and the pro-

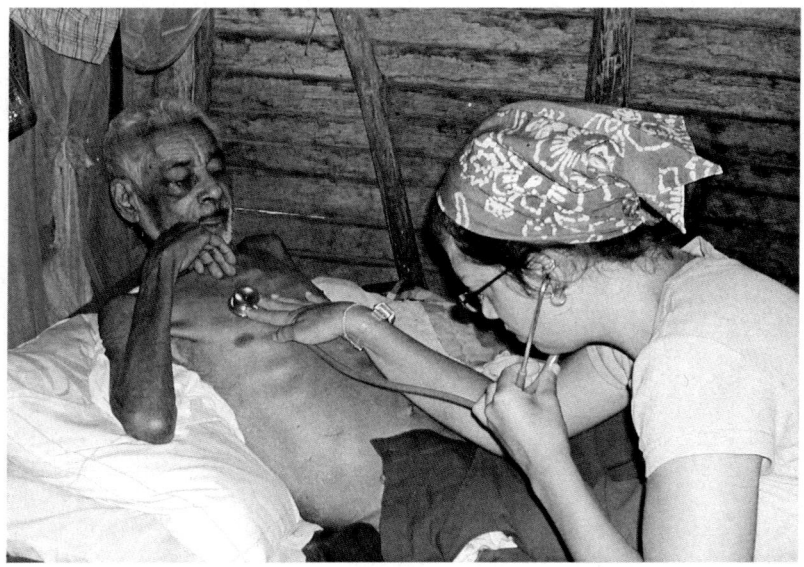

"A religiously inspired principle of healing might be stated this way: the greater the vulnerability of a human being, the greater the protection we ought to afford."
Photographer: Terry Wilwerding

motion of justice should not only define the educational activities of Jesuit colleges and universities. This paradigm should likewise guide the research and service missions as well as the organizational and administrative structures of the schools.

As the many reports that preceded and followed the 2000 Santa Clara conference show, it is not easy to meet the challenging agenda outlined by Father Kolvenbach. Although a remarkable number of programs either were in place or being planned, particularly in the area of education, there is still a long way to go. Too many of these activities are the result of efforts by individual faculty, staff or administrators driven by their own faith and enthusiasm. Little is structural and systemic. For too long a time, Jesuit universities have been busy trying to prove to the outside world that they are on a par with their secular sister institutions or even with the illustrious Ivy League schools. But unlike the great Protestant universities that believed it necessary to shed their religious identity altogether in order to be great institutions of learning, there are still hope and promise for the Jesuit education. After all, the Jesuits are themselves proof that it is certainly possible to be both faithfully committed to a more just world *and* an excellent scientist and scholar.

Still, the challenge is formidable. Historically, Jesuit schools and universities were not founded with the specific intent of educating lay people to become men and women for others. The original Jesuit schools in the Old World were founded to educate future Jesuits. The 28 Jesuit colleges and universities in the New World were founded to offer American Catholics access to quality higher education in a world that was dominated by discriminating and proselytizing Protestant schools. But this threat to the Catholic faith is long gone. Catholics have equal access to public schools. Those schools, by virtue of their secular identity, do not concern themselves with issues of faith. At the dawn of the 21th century, many have asked why the Society of Jesus should nevertheless continue to sponsor colleges and universities. That question has now been answered—at least partially so—in terms of educating for justice. But this answer is in dire need of being systemically operalitionalized—indeed a challenging task.

Nowhere is this challenge more formidable than in the health sciences programs and schools. There are more than 50 health sciences degree programs offered collectively by US Jesuit institutions and many more elsewhere in the world. Our own Creighton University, located in Omaha, Nebraska, alone offers degrees in medicine, dentistry, pharmacy, nursing, occupational therapy, physical therapy, emergency medical services, dental hygiene, biomedical sciences and health administration. Remarkably, only a small number of health sciences delegates were among the several hundred university representatives involved in the national project leading up to the 2000 Santa Clara conference self-study.

One can speculate as to what led to this under representation—and one of us (Welie) has done so in another contribution to this volume.

A Matter of Identity

The fact is that health sciences faculty and administrators have not received much help in figuring out what exactly it means to be a Jesuit health sciences program. Ever since Ignatius excluded schools of medicine and law, deeming such disciplines "more remote" from the Society's formative program, the history of Jesuit health sciences education has been most notable for its silence in the literature. For example, the *Jesuit Educational Quarterly* was published for 32 years (1938-1970). Yet none of its more than 120 issues contains an article on this topic.

This volume is an attempt partially to remedy this problem. The fact that virtually nothing has been written is problematic, but it is also an opportunity. It is an invitation to be creative, to take the heritage of Ignatius and to interpret it anew. If Ignatius were to visit one of the many Jesuit medical centers at the dawn of the 21st century, would he still consider health sciences education "more remote" to the educational mission of the Society? In view of the dramatic injustices in present-day medicine and health care worldwide, but even in economically prosperous countries, we speculate he would not. But what exactly would he expect us to do?

Unfortunately, there is little chance that Ignatius will come to guide us. In this book, a small contingent of Jesuits, lay faculty members and administrators have tried to speak on Ignatius' behalf—a rather arrogant endeavor but one that we may not shun. Indeed, we invite all faculty members and administrators in health sciences degree programs and schools at Jesuit colleges and universities to join in this discussion. This book is aptly subtitled "An Invitation to a Discussion," because the authors are well-aware that their contributions are only a beginning, a first try at best.

We have organized the contributions to this volume in four parts. Part I covers in more general terms the theme of Jesuit education in the 21st century (chapters by Peck and Kolvenbach) and includes a review of the concept of the "preferential option for the poor" (chapter by Massaro). Part II contains three chapters (by Burghardt, Welie and Stempsey) that specifically address the role of Jesuit health sciences programs in promoting justice. Part III contains nine examples of projects that endeavor to teach about justice in health care. We should note that these were not selected by us, the editors, but the result of an invitation by us to all US Jesuit universities to contribute to this volume. In Part IV, three senior administrators (Cristobal, Piront and Davis) from Jesuit health sciences centers share their insights. We close with a bibliography of publications on Jesuit involvement in health care and health sciences throughout the centuries.

Finally, as editors, we wish to dedicate this volume to one of our great teachers, the late David Thomasma, one of the founders of American bioethics. Even though Dave spent most of his academic career at a Jesuit medical center (Loyola University Stritch School of Medicine), few people will associate his work with the project of Jesuit education. And yet we suspect that he would readily agree that Jesuit health sciences education and research ought to be about compassion and justice.

He also knew that education for justice poses a challenging endeavor. Justice is a demanding virtue, as is aptly captured by these quotes from the book *Helping and Healing*, coauthored with his longtime friend and colleague, Edmund Pellegrino:

> A religiously inspired principle of healing might be stated this way: the greater the vulnerability of a human being, the greater the protection we ought to afford. "The first shall be the last, and the last first." This is a derivation from the religious expansion of the principle of justice. In this view, the impediments to equality of respect, in an ideal community, ought to be removed by the members of that community. Civil rights, for example, are a sign of a healing community, not just a set of negotiated entitlements. A healing community must care for those it succors (p. 118)....
>
> [Moreover] in the realms of distributive and social justice, a Christocenric ethic would, of necessity, favor some interpretations of justice over others. Thus, Nozick's fundamental principle of protecting the inequalities of the natural lottery would be the antithesis of a Christian perspective. The Christian vocation is quite specifically oriented to a charitable redress of the inequities of nature or circumstance. It is, in fact, precisely to the losers in the natural lottery—the sick, the poor, the outcast—that Christ addressed his personal ministry and his Sermon on the Mount. This is the basis for the preferential option for the poor that inspires the best Christian institutions.... Compensatory justice makes amends for injustices in the past. In health care, it would call for extra solicitude

for the poor, for minorities, for those who have not had access to health care, and for those treated badly by the natural lottery.... A preferential option for the poor, the disadvantaged, and all who have been ill favored by history, environment, heredity, or political or social circumstance is a necessary extrapolation of the virtue of Christian charity (p. 155)....

The preferential option for the poor is not simply an "option" for Christians. It is an obligation to choose to care for the poor to a greater extent than that found in secular society (p. 121).

References

Arrupe, P (1973). Address to the attendees of the International Congress of Jesuit alumni in Valencia, Spain, July 31. http://www.sjweb.info/education/documents/arr_men_en.doc (site accessed 7/22/04).

Decrees of the 31st and 32nd General Congregations of the Society of Jesus (1977). St. Louis: Institute of Jesuit Sources.

Daoust, J, SJ, (1999). Faith and justice at the core of Jesuit education: Of kingfishers and dragonflies. Keynote address to the attendees of the Western Regional Conference on Justice Education. http://cms.scu.edu/bannancenter/eventsandconferences/justiceconference/westernconference/daoust.cfm (site accessed 7/22/04).

Pellegrino, ED and Thomasma, DC (1997). *Helping and healing: Religious commitment in health care.* Washington DC: Georgetown University Press.

Part I

The Quest for Identity

2. Kirk Peck

A Historical Perspective on Jesuit Higher Education & a Personal Reflection of a Physical Therapy Professor

> Our purpose in education, then, is to form men and women "for others." The Society of Jesus has always sought to imbue students with values that transcend the goals of money, fame and success. We want graduates who will be leaders concerned about society and the world in which they live. We want graduates who desire to eliminate hunger and conflict in the world and who are sensitive to the need for more equitable distribution of the world's goods. We want graduates who seek to end sexual and social discrimination and who are eager to share their faith with others.
>
> Kolvenbach
> *Jesuit Ministry in Higher Education*

I. Living the Jesuit Mission: A Personal Reflection

The premise of this article is to explore Jesuit higher education in light of its extraordinary history and to share my attempt to integrate the values professed by Ignatius into my vocation as a physical therapist. I begin with an experience I had while teaching in one religion-affiliated institution of higher education and describe how that experience influenced my current position as a faculty member in a Jesuit institution. I then depart briefly from my story in order to provide a more in-depth account of some key historical aspects of Catholic and Jesuit higher education. The chapter will conclude with further commentary regarding my ongoing personal journey, including a final reflection.

My story begins in 1993 when I accepted employment at Clarkson College, a small private Episcopalian-affiliated institution in Omaha, Nebraska. I was hired to develop an academic program offering a physical therapist assistant degree. Previously, I had worked full-time as a clinical physical therapist in a private outpatient orthopedic practice but always had an interest in academic teaching and administration. In addition to developing a professional academic program at Clarkson, I participated in campus-wide ceremonial events held for faculty and students. One ceremony that particularly struck me was known as Student Convocation, conducted to introduce incoming students to the university.

Student Convocation was cosponsored with a local Episcopal church. A priest presided over the ceremony who, along with the usual introductions to academia and church, delivered an often humorous, historical account of the church's existence in Nebraska. The priest also relayed a message about the importance of maintaining the church's long standing relationship with the college. I enjoyed Convocation and believed it was important for students to hear about the founding history of the institution they attended. Frequently I wondered how successful the college had been in nurturing its relationship with the Episcopal church. I was curious as to why that relationship seemed to exist only through infrequent ceremonial gatherings. I also wondered why students were not exposed to more formal religious teachings of the Episcopal church. It seemed reasonable to assume religion-affiliated institutions of higher education should demonstrate their commitment to their sponsoring churches.

In 1989, Clarkson developed a loose affiliation with ten other institutions of higher education that shared a common heritage with the Protestant Episcopal church. The Association of Episcopal Colleges emphasized the "linking of faith and values with learning and service" (Association of Episcopal Colleges, 1997, p. 3). The element of service, however, most forcefully struck my attention and prompted me to explore the service mission at the college and at other institutions.

A Historical Perspective on Jesuit Higher Education

Clarkson College is a primarily teaching institution that places a secondary emphasis on public service through its mission of educating health care providers for the community. Scholarly research runs a distant third in importance. Early in 2000, the Clarkson administration further developed the mission of service to the local community and expressed interest in new ideas that might enhance this effort. I therefore talked with a Clarkson College chaplain and the dean of a local Protestant Episcopal church, expressing interest in exploring connections between the mission of Clarkson and the spirit and function of the church. The Episcopal church, I found, had an extensive history of Christian missionary work with a Native American population in northern Nebraska and South Dakota during the late 1800s. Moreover, Bishop Robert Harper Clarkson was included as one of the few Episcopalians who established the first Christian missions to the Ponca

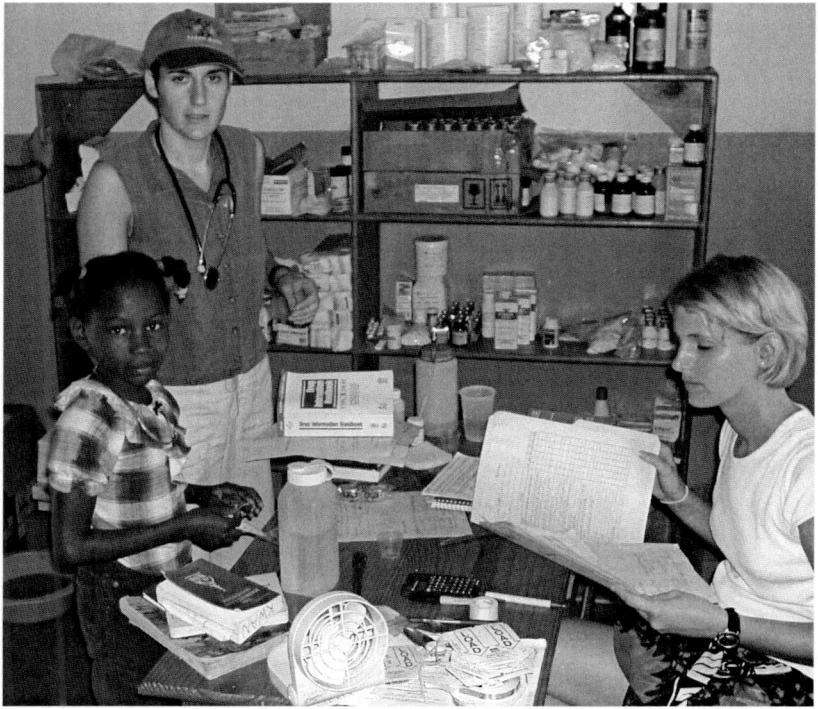

"As we have seen, a pedagogy informed by the *Spiritual Exercises* of Ignatius entails that students . . . learn to discern a call to action."
Photographer: Terry Wilwerding

and Santee Sioux tribes during the 1870s (Barnds, 1969). Members of the tribes exist in Nebraska and South Dakota to this day, and their continued presence facilitated the service connection I sought.

In Nebraska, the Ponca tribe owns a free standing health care clinic, established in 1992, to treat Native Americans from more than seventy tribes. Here, I thought, was a potential link between Clarkson College and the church that could become a meaningful experience for students and faculty alike. Seeing that the relationship would allow the college to share in the church's mission to serve others, I explored a relationship with the Ponca Health care facility. The manager of the Ponca Center was grateful and enthusiastic for the offer of physical therapy services where none were currently available. In the spring of 2000, I established a pro bono physical therapy practice for the Ponca Clinic. The clinic offered both a clinical and cultural service opportunity for both students and faculty. It connected the Episcopal church's belief in service to others and Clarkson College's academic mission to the community. This relationship was unique in that the service I provided as a physical therapist involved a population that has been a part of the Episcopalian missionary effort since its early existence in Nebraska territory. Although I served the Ponca Center on a limited basis (four hours per week), it was still worth my effort since the clinic clientele had no other options for rehabilitative services. The alternative was a seventy-five-mile bus ride from Omaha (Nebraska) to the Winnebago and Macy reservations.

After two wonderful years at the Ponca facility, I accepted a job at a Jesuit university located in Omaha in the spring of 2002. I was particularly drawn to Creighton's historical roots in Jesuit and Catholic philosophy and its mission of service and care for marginalized populations in society. I discussed with the dean of the School of Pharmacy and Health Professions my involvement with Native Americans at the Ponca Center and how it fulfilled my desire to serve underprivileged populations . He assured me that my work was a natural extension of the beliefs and values held by Creighton and encouraged me to continue my efforts as part of the mission of the university. Here I will temporarily depart from my personal story to offer a more in-depth discussion about the importance of connecting values expressed in academic mission statements and those lived experiences found in religion-affiliated institutions of higher education.

II. A Short History of the Mission Debate in Catholic Higher Education

It has long been recognized that nearly all institutions of higher education support a traditional tripartite mission of teaching, research, and service (Johnson, 1997; Veysey, 1965). By virtue of its religious affiliation, a Catholic university adds an additional component, for it is called to "search for the whole truth about nature, man and God" (Pope John Paul II, 1990, p. 1). However, at the dawn of the 21st century, the identity of these Catholic and Jesuit institutions throughout the United States were of widespread concern (Carmody, 2002; Cesareo, 2002; Crowley, 2002; Heft, 1999; Jones, 2002; McMurtrie, 1999; O'Brien, 1994; Kolvenbach, 2001). According to Appleyard and Gray (2000, p. 4), "The conversation about the mission and identity of Jesuit colleges and universities is more than thirty years old and shows no sign of reaching terminal clarity soon." Heft (1999) and Jones (2002) have listed several factors working against the Catholic identity of church-oriented institutions of higher education: (1) an increased secularization of faculty and curriculum; (2) the addition of lay boards of trustees; and (3) a decrease in the number of religious serving in faculty and administrative positions. Experts have responded to this situation by renewed interest in the original intent of the Jesuit mission. Appleyard and Gray (2000) contend that Jesuit higher education evolved through three distinct models of growth over the last thirty years: (1) the control model, (2) the professional model, and (3) the mission model (p. 13).

(1) Following WW II, Jesuit education was characterized by a "control model," in which decisions about governance, curriculum, policy and student formation came from the top down (p. 11). Questions about identity and mission were minimal as it was assumed the Jesuit presence simply took care of these matters. But during the late 1960s and 1970s, several religious communities from universities such as Notre Dame and St. Louis University divested themselves of the

fiduciary responsibility for their institutions. Because many Catholic institutions experienced financial hardships, boards of trustees were reorganized to include lay members with legal and financial expertise. This shift to lay boards was furthered by the decreasing numbers of priests, brothers and sisters in the academies. Administrative control shifted to non-clergy and non-Catholic personnel. The move toward lay boards may also be explained by the Second Vatican Council's (1962-1965) urging that Catholic colleges and universities "[share] governance with the laity" (Heft, 1999, p. 1). Catholic institutions no longer were required to operate under the sole authority of the religion—a signal that even the Vatican was beginning to loosen its hold on institutions of higher education.

The examples of Notre Dame and St. Louis University set a precedent for all Catholic, and thereby Jesuit, institutions to move away from a highly centralized system of administrative control. To some degree, these shifts were appropriate because of concerns about receiving federal and state aid. However, the changes also initiated an even greater secularization and loss of Catholic identity (Appleyard & Gray, 2002).

Lay boards of trustees, however, were not the only force driving institutions toward greater secularization. The Vietnam War, the civil rights movement, social psychology, rock and roll and an increased use of drugs all contributed to the social debate about the Catholic identity of higher education. Traditional differences in attitudes between Catholics and non-Catholics became blurred as Catholics "dabbled in New Age spirituality, got divorces, and disapproved of abortion but accepted the idea that it should be a free choice" (Appleyard & Gray, 2002, p. 5). Many institutions stopped requiring student attendance at mass, mitigated dress codes and stopped separating the genders.

(2) As a result of these changes in church and society, Jesuit schools exchanged the traditional "control model" for a "professional model" (Appleyard & Gray, 2002, p. 12). Institutions realized that survivability in higher education required gaining national recognition for quality research and scholarly activity. Hiring of faculty now hinged more on professional achievements than on staunch support for the Catholic faith. Faculty became increasingly interested in their respective local and national professional organizations than on the

Catholic mission. The gap between church philosophy and professional recognition grew. Appleyard and Gray conclude: "Moreover, then as now, faculty professional ethos was very different from that of administration and staff; the latter tended to support institutional identity as a matter of course, whereas the former put a high priority on academic freedom, self-governance, and a faculty role in making academic policy-values not every Catholic institution was used to endorsing" (2002, p. 6). Requirements for core curricula were reduced or eliminated altogether, and faculty advisement centered more on academic issues than on personal formation. Cesarao (2002) has labeled this approach as a "secular model" of education (p. 26). Professional studies and academic disciplines dominated curriculum, sacrificing courses on Catholic philosophy.

Responding to the lay boards in the late 1960s, the Association of Catholic Colleges and Universities insisted that it is "the final responsibility of the boards of trustees to maintain the Catholic character of the institutions" (Jones, 2002, p. 3). Convening at Land O'Lakes Wisconsin in 1967, educators issued a document acknowledging that "The Catholic university must have a true autonomy and academic freedom in the face of authority of whatever kind, lay or clerical, external to the academic community." However, "A Catholic institution must be a community in which Catholicism is perceptibly present and effectively operative" (Heft, 1999, p. 1). The document supported the Vatican II Council but also reinforced the importance of colleges' and universities' Catholic identity, despite the pressing internal and external forces.

But more than 25 years after the Land O'Lakes conference, the identity crisis in Catholic higher education is not resolved. Referencing historian Philip Gleason, O'Brien concluded that the assimilation of Catholic institutions to secular norms has only gathered momentum. He expressed concern that "Catholic colleges and universities were in danger of repeating the history of once-Protestant schools that gradually threw off their church affiliation, moved religion out of a serious role in academic life, and ended up as secular institutions with no particular religious identity" (1994, p. 97).

(3) As a result of calls for a renewed focus on identity and mission, in the nineteen-nineties the "mission model" emerged (Appleyard

& Gray, 2002, p. 13). Now administrators and educators refocused attention on the founding principles of Jesuit education that sought to develop students by integrating social context with professional development and commitment. Philosophically, this model diminished the importance of the professional model and asked the question, "How do faith and learning mutually challenge and enrich each other?" (Appleyard & Gray, 2002, p. 13). Appleyard and Gray conclude that Jesuit education, by incorporating the mission model, will produce "not just knowledge, skills, and cultural savvy but also a depth of reflection, maturity, and spiritual character that marks the way its graduates approach the world" (2002, p. 13). Carmody adds, "A diploma from a Catholic university should equip and motivate the recipient to grow into the fullness of her or his humanity" (2002, p. 5).

Cesareo cites institutions that incorporate programs focused on Catholic studies and that preserve a unique mission and identity. Moreover, he insists that Catholic studies "are the responsibility of every member of the university or college community—regardless of specialty, discipline, or background—to ensure that Catholicism is vitally present and operative" (2002, p. 30).

These authors are aware that the adoption of a mission model is not likely to receive institution-wide support. After all, "Mission is rooted in our fundamental religious values, not in creedal conformity" (Carmody, 2002, p. 7). Carmody predicts that institutions seeking to adopt such a model may be charged with "changing direction, losing intellectual commitment, pandering to liberal propaganda, becoming shills for the hierarchy, or caving in to the administration or to some segment of the faculty, staff, or student body." Moreover, "Possibly the most often-voiced criticism will be that we are hypocritical" (p. 7).

III. The Vatican Response to Catholic Identity

A thorough exploration of the Vatican's involvement with Catholic higher education is beyond the scope of this contribution; however, we must look at selected related documents. In 1972, *The Catholic University in the Modern World* was published by a congress of Catholic universities. It outlined four characteristics shared by all Catholic institutions of higher education: (1) a Christian inspiration of the academic community; (2) a continuing reflection, in light of the Catholic faith, upon the expansion of human knowledge; (3) a fidelity to the Christian message as it comes through the church; and (4) a commitment to the service of the church, to all humanity and to the transcendent meaning of life (Heft, 1999, p. 2). The Congress reiterated that even institutions not chartered by the Holy See were accountable to these four characteristics. Confusion, however, remained as to the limits of authority the church held over non-pontifically chartered schools.

A revised copy of the *Roman Catholic Code of Canon Law* in 1983 reaffirmed the authority of the church to create and govern universities. It stated that faculty should be "outstanding in their integrity of doctrine and uprightness of life"; desired that theologians receive a mandate from the church to teach Catholic doctrine; and wanted university presidents to take an oath of faith to the church (Heft, 1999, p. 2; Wilson, 2001). Debate on church authority over non-pontifically established institutions continued until 1990, when the Holy See was issued a new document, *Ex Corde Ecclesiae* (Heft, 1999). It applied to institutions throughout the world (National Conference of Catholic Bishops, 2000). The Holy See declared that "A Catholic university, as Catholic, is linked with the church either through a formal, constitutive and statutory bond or by reason of an institutional commitment made by those responsible for it" (Pope John Paul II, 1990, p. 8). In addition, the document stated that bishops, "even when they do not enter directly into the internal governance of the university, should be seen not as external agents but as participants in the life of the Catholic university (Pope John Paul II, 1990, p. 5). It urged each university to "hire a majority of Catholic faculties, appoint a majority of Catholic trustees and elect Catholic presidents" (Pope John Paul II, 1990). Jesuit universities, as other Catholic institutions, abide by *Ex Corde Ecclesiae*. The goals of Jesuit universities and the church are harmonized by administrators reflection upon issues such as academic curriculum, faculty hiring practices and governing authority. Faculties in Jesuit institutions need to remain flexible in response to administrative needs while remain vigilant to their autonomy regarding academic freedom in the classroom.

The document drew significant criticism. Wilson warned universities and church authorities alike to be prudent when discussing the legal ramifications of the application of *Ex Corde Ecclesiae*. After all, *Ex Corde Ecclesiae* has "no legally binding effect on Catholic colleges and universities, unless institutional governing boards expressly adopt them" (2001, p. 2). According to civil law, universities maintain a right to adopt *Ex Corde Ecclesiae* in its entirety, modify it through governing board authority or reject the document outright. In addition, universities electing to adopt *Ex Corde Ecclesiae* in full or with modifications must amend all institutional governing documents accordingly (Wilson, 2001). Governing documents include faculty handbooks, institutional bylaws and, in some cases, faculty contracts.

In spite of potential legal ramifications, the majority of Catholic colleges and universities have maintained a positive view of *Ex Corde Ecclesiae* (Moser, 2002). Referencing a quotation by Sister Karen Kennelly, former president of Mount, St. Mary's in Los Angeles, Moser equates the document to "a 'call' to promote dialogue between faith and culture, between faith and reason" (2002, p. 21). Indeed, it has many advocates (Heft, 1999). Some experts have viewed *Ex corde* as a partial panacea for two reasons. First, the document involved Catholic institutions' renewal of their ties to the church, thus counteracting the pressure of secularization. Second, the document mandated that curricula remain in accordance with church doctrine. The mandate stymied theologians who openly countered church teaching (Heft, 1999).

Ex Corde Ecclesiae is not simply aimed at establishing authority over universities. Rather the document acknowledges the importance of universities for the church, as evidenced by its title that literally translated means "from the heart of the church." It describes both the mission and identity and outlines the Holy See's expectations for colleges and universities in fulfilling their academic missions. The "Apostolic Constitution on Catholic Universities" is a call for universities to renew their identities as both "universities" and "Catholic" and outlines their four characteristics:

> (1) Christian inspiration not only of individuals but of the university community as such; (2) a continuing reflection in the light of the Catholic faith upon the growing treasury of human knowledge, to

which it seeks to contribute by its own research; (3) fidelity to the Christian message as it comes to us through the church; and (4) an institutional commitment to the service of the people of God and of the human family in their pilgrimage to the transcendent goal which gives meaning to life (Pope John Paul II, 1990, pp. 2-3).

According to Lannon (2001), "The issue facing both the leaders of American Catholic higher education and the bishops is locating a balance where the Catholic university is faithful to both the values of American higher education and Catholic identity" (p. 36). His findings support presidents at Jesuit universities in promoting Catholic mission and identity. But to maintain or restore an identity where it has been either blurred or lost requires more than rhetoric from a college president. Faculty also need to be a vital part of the process (Feeney, Gilman & Parker, 1997; Passon, 1997).

Appropriately, *Ex Corde Ecclesiae* underscores the importance of faculty in institutions of higher education. In "Article 4: The University Community," says that all professors "at the time of their appointment, are to be informed about the Catholic identity of the institution and its implications, and about their responsibility to promote, or at least to respect, that identity." It further stresses that "In ways appropriate to different academic disciplines, all Catholic teachers are to be faithful to, and all other teachers are to respect, Catholic doctrine and morals in their research and teaching" (Pope John Paul II, 1990, p. 9). In an effort to apply these norms, proceedings from the National Conference of Catholic Bishops state that "When these qualities are suspect or lacking, the university statutes are to specify the competent authority and the process to be followed to remedy the situation" (National Conference of Catholic Bishops, 2000, p. 15). This declaration stresses the need for faculty to be aware of and in tune with the mission and values of the church. Therefore, faculty at Jesuit universities must acquire a sound understanding and appreciation of the rich history of Jesuit education as originally envisioned by its founder and since expanded by generations of Jesuit and lay educators.

IV. Early Jesuit Education

Historically, Jesuit institutions have been successful in fulfilling the standards of a university while remaining Catholic and Jesuit. Morrison has described a Jesuit university in relation to three characteristics: Jesuit institutions are (1) universities by offering "diverse programs, expanding in offerings and striving constantly for the highest excellence in all endeavors" (1995, p. 10); (2) Catholic by maintaining a "commitment to the Catholic tradition and ideals," in other words, "Catholic in inspiration" (p. 28); and (3) Jesuit in respect for the long tradition and history of the Society of Jesus and through the spirituality illuminated by Ignatius's *Spiritual Exercises* that "create a drive to know, a drive to be educated, a drive to teach others about the realities that God has given us in his loving plan" (p. 18).

The first Jesuit school of education was founded by Ignatius in Messina, Sicily, in 1548. The school was established to provide an education for lay students known as "externs" with the purpose of training young men to become "catechists, preachers, and evangelists" (Maher, Shore & Parker, 1999; O'Malley, 1999; O'Malley, 2000). Ignatius never intended to establish formalized educational programs as a part of the original Jesuit mission. However, he soon realized that students who acquired Jesuit training were the best prepared to serve society as civic and religious leaders throughout the world and to spread the philosophy of the Jesuit tradition on a global scale (Holy Cross, 2002; Kolvenbach, 1989; Kolvenbach, 2001; Maher, Shore & Parker, 1999; O'Malley, 1999; The Jesuit Community, 2002). Subjects such as drama, art, music and opera were introduced early in the curriculum to provide students with a sense of culture and well-roundedness (Modras, 2000). Having received requests to begin schools in other parts of Europe, Ignatius sent a letter to the king of Portugal acknowledging Jesuit education had become one of the best mechanisms for spreading the faith. Ignatius wrote:

> I have come to the conclusion that the service of men and thus the glory of God our Lord will be furthered in that Kingdom if the members of our Society were to make it their business to open schools where young people can be taught virtue and letters and

their parents and households drawn closer to God through them (Coleman, 2002, p. 2).

By 1551, Ignatius had opened the Roman College with additional Jesuit schools being founded in Vienna and Palermo. By the time of Ignatius's death in 1556, the number of Jesuit schools had reached thirty-five (O'Malley, 1999; O'Malley, 2000; The Loyola institute, 2002). They continued to grow in number until 1773, when, by papal order, the Society of Jesus was abolished. The network of schools, consisting of more than eight hundred universities, seminaries and other schools spread throughout Europe, Asia and Africa, was disbanded. In 1814, Pope Pius VII realized the benefit Jesuit education brought to the church and restored the Jesuit order. Though many schools and colleges were never reopened, the rebuilt network has remained one of the largest educational systems ever developed (The Loyola Institute, 2002).

V. Ignatian Spirituality, the Spiritual Exercises, and Jesuit Education

The philosophy of Jesuit education largely was influenced by Ignatius's experiences with the *Spiritual Exercises* with the ultimate goal of the Exercises to "glorify God" (Coleman 1997, p. 2). "Spirituality" is an equivocal term, used in multiple ways that are frequently confounding or even misguided. The term is often used interchangeably with "religion," increasing the confusion. According to Tisdell (2001), "Religion is an organized community of faith that has written codes of regulatory behavior, whereas spirituality is more about one's personal belief and experience of a higher power or higher purpose" (p.1).

The form of spirituality that is supposed to pervade Jesuit higher education is not just any kind, but Ignatian spirituality, largely derived from the prayer and meditation one experiences through the *Spiritual Exercises*. Downey defines "Christian spirituality," of which the Ignatian version is part, as both a "lived experience and an academic discipline," reflecting a "whole of the Christian's life as this is oriented to self-transcending knowledge, freedom, and love in light of the ultimate values and highest ideals perceived and pursued in the mystery of Jesus Christ through the Holy Spirit in the church, and the community of disciplines" (1991, p. 1). Basing himself on Ignatius, Padberg characterizes Ignatian spirituality by listing a series of characteristics: "experience and reflective discernment of that experience, discernment followed by action, service of the needy and cultivation of the powerful, individuality and community, spontaneity and organization, initiative and divestment, Jesuits and others as companions in following in love with the example of Christ, the human common good and the infinite majesty of God (for Ignatius best expressed in his ardent devotion to the Holy Trinity), finding God in all things and accommodation or adaptation to the real circumstances in which this spirituality was to be lived out" (1999, pp. 2-3).

Shortly after his conversion, Ignatius embarked on a pilgrimage during which he visited, and remained at, the shrine of our Lady at Montserrat. For the following ten months, Ignatius lived as a hermit in nearby Manresa praying and doing penance (Walsh, 1991). During his hermitage, Ignatius recorded in a journal his thoughts on spirituality and on his personal transformation. These reflections would become known as the *Spiritual Exercises* (McBrien, 2001).

The final version of the *Spiritual Exercises* resulted after fifteen years of refinement and was first published after papal approval in 1548. They reflect Ignatius's understanding of an orderly process for spiritual development (Callahan, 1997). As a result of political controversy over the book's publication, he was tried for heresy during the Spanish Inquisition (Walsh, 1991). Never convicted, he served time in jail while his book of *Exercises* was examined by court authorities (McBrien, 2001). After surviving the Inquisition, his *Spiritual Exercises* flourished for the next 450 years, but not without being subjected to frequent reinterpretation. Despite continuous critiques, the book has remained the key source of inspiration for defining Jesuit spirituality and describing the philosophy of Ignatian pedagogy (Coleman, 2002; Day & Scroope, 2002; Kolvenbach, 1998; International Center for Jesuit Education, 2002; Sharkey, 2002).

Callahan argues that the *Spiritual Exercises* were intended to be a guide book for a "series of spiritual activities" and it is a "book to be done, rather than a book to be read" (1997). The *Exercises* are about "choice and decision-making" with a "thrust towards action, not simply reflection." In addition, the *Exercises* are meant to bring about an inner "balance" allowing one to enjoy freedom of decision-making based on an acquired knowledge of values in tune with God. The relevance of the *Spiritual Exercises* for education is clear. They are "more than a method of personal growth in the spiritual life. Their world view and methods became the foundation upon which the whole system of Jesuit education was built" (Callahan 1997). Key pedagogical characteristics have emerged from the *Exercises* as a manifestation of Ignatian spirituality, specifically experience, reflection, and action, about which more shall be said in a subsequent section.

VI. Towards a "Well-ordered" Plan: The *Ratio Studiorum*

Jesuit philosophy proclaims that one should seek to "find God in all things" and to do so with a "well-ordered plan" (Maher, Shore & Parker, 1999, p. 48). This philosophy applies to all of the Society's missions, including education. Although such a "well ordered plan" for Jesuit education would only be developed several decades after Ignatius' death (see below for a discussion of the *Ratio Studiorum*), Ignatius' own experiences as a student at several universities and particularly at the University of Paris, influenced his plans for the newly established schools. Ignatius began his formal studies in Alcala, Spain. Frustrated with a lack of organization, however, traveled to Paris where he was introduced to a system known as the "modus Parisiensis" (Cordina, 2000, p. 38). At the University of Paris, he studied medieval scholasticism (Matthews & Platt, 1992). Regardless of age, students were divided into separate classes based solely on an entrance exam. They were not allowed to progress to a higher level of studies without first passing lower course exams. Instructional methodology was broken into periods of lecture, questions from instructors and disputations or debates to facilitate understanding of course material. The students were presented with a problem; they argued for and against the issue using ancient authors such as Aristotelian writings, church doctrine and the Bible. They then offered a solution to the problem from the sources (Matthews & Platt, 1992).

In addition to extensive educational experiences in the university, Ignatius's philosophy of learning was influenced by the onset of Renaissance humanism. During the later half of the fifteenth and into the early sixteenth century, Greek and Latin classics reemerged. The University of Paris, like many other colleges, adopted the newfound interest in humanistic education characterized by study of the classical languages, grammar, rhetoric and the arts (Codina, 2000; Graves, 1926).

Ignatius' commitment to humanistic education became one of the hallmarks of the Jesuit order for the next 450 years (Chittister, 2001). He determined the basic guidelines for the organization of these institutions in the Part IV of the Society's Constitutions. In it, he stressed the importance of acquiring a well-rounded education founded in the humanities, philosophy and theology. However, this part of the Constitutions left much to be developed regarding specifics of educational rules and regulations. Ignatius had hoped to create a set of rules to govern Jesuit schools such as those at the Roman College but failed to achieve this goal before his death in 1556 (The Loyola Institute, 2002).

In 1599, 43 years after his death, a more elaborate document on Jesuit education, the *Ratio Studiorum*, or "plan of studies," established the philosophical foundation and model of early Jesuit education, which would undergo little variation until 1832. At that time, mathematics, natural science, history and geography were added to the curriculum without sacrificing the classics (Graves, 1926).

The *Ratio Studiorum* was written by Father General Claudio Aquaviva, then Superior General of the Society of Jesus, creating a manual suitable for Jesuit instruction (Harvanek, 1989). The *Ratio* contained four key elements: (1) students were required to gain a basic knowledge of Greek language and rhetoric; (2) instructors were to educate students about values and attitudes reflective of Jesuit thought; (3) a strong emphasis was placed on engaging students in the learning process along with a continuous evaluation of their progress; (4) students should obtain a certain level of knowledge and abilities before progressing with their studies (Maher, Shore & Parker, 1999). The primary purpose of the

Ratio, however, was "to instill knowledge and love of the creator and redeemer of humanity" (Maher, Shore & Parker, 1999, p. 50).

Unquestionably, the *Ratio's* structure and organization were important to the Society of Jesus in the sixteenth and seventeenth centuries. O'Malley (1999) has described it as the "Magna Carta" of Jesuit education because it included a required curriculum. It accomplished Ignatius' vision that Jesuit education be a "well ordered progress of studies," and it flourished as one of the best and most highly structured and organized set of principles ever outlined for formalized education (Maher, Shore & Parker, 1999, p. 48). But the *Ratio* was not to persist in its original form forever. With the passing of time, Jesuit universities ultimately rode the wave of secularization along with other Catholic universities (Appleyard & Gray, 2000; Crowley, 2002; Duminuco, 2000; Kolvenbach, 2001; O'Brien, 1994).

VII. Contemporary Ignatian Pedagogy

The expansion of boards to include lay members, diminishing numbers of Jesuits on campuses and a relaxed religious authority within Jesuit universities have all contributed to a present-day crises of Jesuit identity (McMurtrie, 1999). Crowley observed that "Perhaps the fundamental problem facing Jesuit education today, the one problem underlying all the others, is primarily a problem of spirituality, of a search for transcendence" (2002, p. 10). Many Jesuit institutions have succumbed to the "complications and seductions of power, big money, and prestige" which is in direct conflict with a simultaneous desire to "recover the identity of the Jesuit educational tradition" (p. 10).

Concerns for a contemporary version of Jesuit mission and identity in secondary education motivated former Superior General Father Pedro Arrupe to establish the International Commission on the Apostolate of Jesuit Education in 1980. After several years of deliberation, one of the most widely distributed documents in Jesuit history was issued. The 1986 document, *The Characteristics of Jesuit Education*, was made available to Jesuit institutions, including a translation into thirteen languages (Duminuco, 2000). The document outlined nine primary characteristics of Jesuit education, including extensive commentary.

Although the *Characteristics* were primarily intended for secondary education, Arrupe's successor Father Peter Hans Kolvenbach has asserted that the document was "applicable to all areas of Jesuit education" (Duminuco, 2000, p. 152).

Jesuit education, according to this document:

1. Is world-affirming, assisting in the total formation of each individual within the human community. It includes a religious dimension that permeates the entire education and it is an apostolic instrument, promoting dialogue between faith and culture.

2. Insists on individual care and concern for each person, emphasizing activity on the part of the student and encouraging lifelong openness to growth.

3. Is value-oriented, encouraging a realistic knowledge, love and acceptance of self and providing a realistic knowledge of the world in which we live.

4. Proposes Christ as the model of human life. It provides adequate pastoral care, celebrating faith in personal and community prayer, worship and service.

5. Is preparation for active life commitment, serving the faith that does justice. It seeks to form "men and women for others," manifesting a particular concern for the poor.

6. Is an apostolic instrument, in service of the church as it serves human society. It prepares students for active participation in the church and the local community, for the service of others.

7. Pursues excellence in its work of formation and witnesses to excellence.

8. Stresses lay-Jesuit collaboration relying on a spirit of community among teaching staff and administrators, the Jesuit community, governing boards, parents, former students and benefactors. It takes place within a structure that promotes community.

9. Adapts means and methods in order to achieve its purposes most effectively. It is a "system" of schools with a common vision and common goals, assisting in providing the professional training and ongoing formation that is needed, especially for teachers (Duminuco, 2000, pp. 168-211; The Loyola Institute, 2002).

Faculty and administrators were pleased with the outcome of the *Characteristics* in helping to "clarify the nature and mission of Jesuit schools" (Duminuco, 2000, p. 153). Following three years of implementation, however, one question remained: "In order to realize the goals, to make the principles take life, how can we make the characteristics real in the daily interaction between teacher and student, so that we can move from theory into practice, from rhetoric into reality" (p. 153)? The seriousness of this question put the International Commission on the Apostolate of Jesuit Education to the task and by 1993 the Commission produced a document, changing Jesuit education once again. A document titled *Ignatian Pedagogy: a Practical Approach* provided educators with a template for the instruction long envisioned by Ignatius himself (Duminuco, 2000; International Center for Jesuit Education, 2002).

Sharkey (2002) describes Ignatian pedagogy as "a process whereby teachers can promote the Jesuit mission in the classes they teach and in the various other ways in which they are engaged with their students." *"Ignatian Pedagogy* is the formation of students who are leaders in service, in imitation of Christ Jesus, men and women of competence, conscience and compassionate commitment" (p. 2). Central to this thought about student development are the three concepts establishing the initial hallmarks of Ignatian pedagogy: experience, reflection and action. In order to make it more contemporary, two additional elements were added: context and evaluation" (The Loyola Institute, 2002, p. 1; International Center for Jesuit Education, 2002). Context would mark the initial aspect underlying the philosophy of Ignatian pedagogy while evaluation would conclude the process.

(1) Context. Instructors need to become as familiar as possible with the students being taught. Context, in this case, referred to a background knowledge of each student in relation to family, friends, culture, socioeconomic status, religious beliefs and other past learning experiences (Sharkey, 2002; International Center for Jesuit Education, 2002). Requiring instructors to learn about their students stems from the process used in giving the Spiritual Exercises. For instance, to assess the readiness for the Exercises, Ignatius began by learning all he could about the subject's personality and experiences. The key to such discovery, for Ignatius, was to gain assurance that a retreatant was serious about meditating on God (International Center for Jesuit Education, 2002).

(2) Experience. In giving the Spiritual Exercises, Ignatius sought to engage the "whole person" in the learning experience. This included not only intellectual ability but also, as Ignatius put it, "to taste something internally" (International Center for Jesuit Education, 2002, §42). The key to "experience" was to get students to "feel something about what they learn if they are going to end up doing something about it." The accumulation of knowledge and rote memorization was not enough. Their "intellectual grasp" of a topic had to be joined to "an internal feeling" (Sharkey, 2002, p.3). In other words, students were to have an emotional or affective response to their learning if they were to be moved to action.

(3) Reflection. Father Kolvenbach, the present Superior General of the Society, has emphasized that "we must exercise discernment, which implies asking questions, searching for solutions, learning from experience and research" if we are to differentiate good from bad (2002, p. 4). Applied to Ignatian pedagogy, discernment means "clarifying internal motivation" (p. 4). Expanding on the concept of "experience" described earlier, "reflection" is defined as a "thoughtful consideration of some subject matter, experience, idea, purpose or spontaneous reaction, in order to grasp its significance more fully" (International Center for Jesuit Education, 2002, §49). Therefore, a student must reflect upon inner emotional reactions to things and ideas learned in order to fully grasp the value of their education. Without reflection, learning is void of meaning. Reflection on a past experience is a way of "validating its authenticity" (§25).

(4) Action. According to Ignatius, "Love is shown in deeds, not words" (International Center for Jesuit Education, 2002, §59). The same adage applied to education. Experience and reflection are key elements but hold little meaning unless there is a subsequent call to action. Action is based on an integration of the cognitive and affected reactions to experience and the meanings and values extrapolated from experience through the process of reflection (International Center for Jesuit Education, 2002). Action has to be both "interiorized and externally manifested" (Sharkey, 2002, p. 4). Interiorized choices occur when students take to heart what they have learned through experience and reflection and commit their life to what they perceived as truth. In time, students externalize the commitment to truth and are com-

pelled "to act, to do something consistent with this new conviction" (International Center for Jesuit Education, 2002, §62).

(5) Evaluation. The final step of Ignatian pedagogy is the process of evaluation. Although not part of the original philosophy of the Spiritual Exercises, Ignatian pedagogy has always recognized that "periodic evaluation of the student's growth in attitudes, priorities and actions consistent with being a person for others is essential" (International Center for Jesuit Education, 2002, §64). Examples include "mentoring, review of student journals, student self-evaluation in light of personal growth profiles, as well as review of leisure time activities and voluntary service to others" (International Center for Jesuit Education, 2002, §65).

Taken together, the five elements of context, experience, reflection, action and evaluation characterize the Jesuit philosophy of education. The overall goal of Ignatian education is to develop a "well-rounded" student. But such education is always a process, instilling "lifelong habits of learning that foster attention to experience, reflective understanding beyond self-interest, and criteria for responsible action" (International Center for Jesuit Education, 2002, §70). If successful, the student will mature into a person

- who will gradually learn to discriminate and be selective in choosing experiences;
- who is able to draw fullness and richness from the reflection on those experiences; and
- who becomes self-motivated by his or her own integrity and humanity to make conscious, responsible choices. (International Center for Jesuit Education, 2002, §69)

Of course, all of this can only come about if faculty and administrators at Jesuit universities are committed to the Ignatian pedagogy, which in turn assumes that they are knowledgeable about it. In a 1989 address, Superior General Father Kolvenbach argued, first, that the "distinctive role of the Jesuits in a Jesuit university is to share the basic Ignatian purpose and thrust of Jesuit education." Second, "it is an obligation in justice to acquaint prospective administrators, professors and staff with the spirit of the institution and to ask if they can share in its spirit and contribute to its mission." Thus, if the Jesuit mission is to be revitalized, there must be a physical presence and interaction with Jesuits on campus in order to properly transmit the "values of Jesuit education and the spirituality from which they flow," and faculty, staff and administrators must share a common understanding if they are to successfully espouse the Jesuit mission. (Callahan, 1998, p. 11) Spoken at Georgetown University, Kolvenbach's instructions apply to all Jesuit universities.

VIII. Living the Jesuit Mission: Creighton University

Creighton University, located in Omaha, Nebraska, is one of twenty-eight Jesuit universities located in the United States. It was founded in 1878 by Mary Lucretia Creighton, the widow of Edward Creighton, an early pioneer of the transcontinental telegraph. It was Edward's wish to establish a university in the Midwest. The Jesuit order has managed the university since its doors first opened (*Creighton University Bulletin,* 2001). Today, Creighton supports an annual enrollment of more than 6,000 students seeking degrees in a variety of disciplines including medicine, dentistry, law, business, education and the arts and sciences. (Creighton University Home Page, 2004).

The mission of the university explicitly embraces the importance of seeking the truth through diversity yet remaining faithful to its Catholic and Jesuit heritage. The mission statement includes the following paragraph:

> As Catholic, Creighton University is dedicated to the pursuit of truth in all its forms and is guided by the living tradition of the Catholic church. As Jesuit, Creighton University participates in the tradition of the Society of Jesus which provides an integrating vision of the world that arises out of a knowledge and love of Jesus Christ. As comprehensive, Creighton University's education embraces several colleges and professional schools and is directed to the intellectual, social, spiritual, physical and recreational aspects of students' lives and to the promotion of justice (*Creighton University Bulletin,* 2001, p.1).

Students at Creighton are not required to participate in on-campus religious services or activities, but a common goal of the institution is to foster a sense of spiritual well-being as a part of developing graduates for the betterment of society. This goal is expressed through the university's identity with the Society of Jesus and its association with the principles and morals of the Catholic faith.

During his inaugural address as the twenty-third president at Creighton University, John P. Schlegel, SJ, reaffirmed the importance of the relationship between the Jesuit mission and that of the Catholic church. According to Schlegel, the university "interprets the church to the world and the world to the church" (2000, p. 5). Those words strengthened the assumption that Creighton is not only an institution espousing the importance of knowledge and wisdom but a center of learning where the academic community and students alike actively seek to explore the true spirit of humanity.

Father Schlegel also emphasized Creighton's relationship to the church by stating: "Creighton University has recognized its special relationship to the Catholic church at both the local and the universal level. In this context of a Catholic university, theology, philosophy, and moral behavior are integral as we provide a setting where religious experience and secular experience join in dialogue to meet the issues of the day" (p.3). To manifest a vision of such dialogue requires faculty to integrate appropriate learning opportunities into respective curricula. As previously described, however, the best mechanism to accomplish this goal remains a challenge for most Jesuit institutions.

IX. Living the Jesuit Mission: A Personal Reflection Continued

In response to Father Schlegel's remarks concerning the relationship between church and academy, I return to my personal reflection on living the Jesuit mission. Shortly after my move from Clarkson College to Creighton University in the spring of 2002, two other persons and I completed an unpublished study as part of my doctoral degree. It explored how faculty members at Creighton, which considers spirituality to be part of its mission, perceive their own responsibility to foster spirituality. Outcomes of the study were intriguing. Faculty members expressed the belief that spirituality, although hard to define, was best fostered through personal actions, faculty role-modeling and integrated course activities. In addition, faculty related the importance of symbolism (e.g., crucifixes in classrooms and an on-campus Catholic parish) as key factors to the expression of spirituality.

The study made me realize the complexity by which faculty interpreted and measured the concept of spirituality. How would faculty have responded if more specifics had been given to the meaning of spirituality at this particular university? In what manner would faculty at a Jesuit university interpret and incorporate the concept of Ignatian spirituality? And more specifically, in what manner do faculty in health science disciplines fulfill the academic mission?

I was motivated to formulate my own answer to the latter question when I first offered physical therapy services to the Native American population prior to taking my position at Creighton. At the time, I had a deep and personal desire to do something for the public good and my primary intention was to use my skills as a physical therapist to provide health care to an underserved population. I had found an accepting environment at the Ponca Center where I not only provided patient care for those in need, but I could fulfill a desire to serve God in a more personal and meaningful way.

I would characterize my motivation to serve a disadvantaged population as a spirituality trying to manifest itself in a humanistic and observable manner. In essence, this form of spiritual discernment, where reflection was followed by action, is much the same as that described by the spirituality of Ignatius. Although my service may or may not be strictly Ignatian, I believe it exemplifies a spirituality compatible with the Christian faith— to treat all humans with respect and dignity and to have compassion and care for the less fortunate. It is embodied in care and concern combined with my personal calling to physical therapy. It is the expression of my spirituality.

Reflecting on my researching the link between mission and service, I am reminded of a passage by Linda Chisholm, past President of the Association of Episcopal Colleges. During an address delivered to the colleges and universities of the Anglican Communion, Dr. Chisholm articulated the link between service and academic mission when she stated, "Service—community, public, human service—is the natural intersection between the church and the college or university" (1993, p. 2). This statement solidified the connecting of mission to action and more importantly of connecting action to the specific values expressed by a religion-affiliated institution's academic mission. Likewise, Creighton by nature of its own academic mission, claims both spirituality and justice as the key elements it its identity. The university has enabled me to fulfill a personal conviction to better society by providing a service through my profession. It has indeed turned my profession into a spiritual vocation— one that parallels Creighton's academic mission.

My work at the Ponca Center contributes, in another unique way to the educational mission of Creighton University. To truly fulfill the academic mission of forming men and women for and with others, students themselves must become actively engaged in the spirited mission of serving others in need. As we have seen, a pedagogy informed by the *Spiritual Exercises* of Ignatius entails that students have an engaged experience, opportunities for a reflection on the experience and learn to discern a call to action (Padberg, 1999). Exposing students to a pedagogy such as this will never occur, however, unless faculty in Jesuit-based universities incorporate explicit examples of this style of education in the courses they teach. Although I feel far from being that ideal example for students, I do carry some comfort in perceiving that at least I have attempted to make a personal difference to society and the academy in a unique and meaningful way.

In the leading quotation of this article, Father Kolvenbach expressed the importance of Creighton's mission to serve others by emphasizing the application of this goal for all Jesuit institutions. "Our purpose in education, then, is to form men and women 'for others'... Graduates will be leaders concerned about society and the world in which they live" and "who desire to eliminate hunger and conflict in the world and who are sensitive to the need for more equitable distribution of the world's goods" (Kolvenbach, 1989). By continuing my work with the Native American population at the Ponca Health and Wellness Center while employed at Creighton University, I have taken the first step towards what I believe is living the Jesuit mission: Serving the underserved and being a role model for students embarking on a professional career in physical therapy in which ideally the Jesuit phrase "the service of faith and promotion of justice" takes personal meaning in the heart of every graduate (Kolvenbach, p. 1, 2000).

References

Appleyard, J & Gray, H (2000). Tracking the mission and identity question: Three decades of inquiry and three models of interpretation. *Conversations,* 18, 4-15.

Association of Episcopal Colleges (1997). *Guide to Episcopal colleges.* Association of Episcopal Colleges: New York: NY.

Barnds, W (1969). *The Episcopal church in Nebraska: A centennial history.* Omaha: Omaha Printing Co.

Burkhardt, M (1989). Spirituality: An analysis of the concept. *Holistic Nursing Practice,* 3, 69-77.

Callahan, J (1997). *Discovering a sacred world: Ignatius of Loyola's Spiritual Exercises and its influence on education.* Kansas City: Rockhurst University. Reprinted by the Jesuits of the Missouri Province, St. Louis, Missouri. www.creighton.edu/Heartland3/r-comingterms.html (site accessed on 10/24/02).

———. (1998). *Coming to terms with the mission: The Catholic and Jesuit university in America.* Kansas City: Rockhurst University. www.rockhurst. edu/about/jesuitheritage/terms.pdf (site accessed July 19, 2004).

Carmody, D (2002). The catholicity of the Catholic university. *Conversations,* 22, 4-Nine.

Cesareo, F (2002). Where knowledge and faith meet: Catholic studies and the questions of identity. *Conversations,* 22, 24-31.

Chisholm, L (1993). Student volunteer services. Speech presented to colleges and universities of the Anglican Communion at Canterbury, England.

Chittister, J (2001). Students and the curriculum in an Ignatian school. Presented at the National Catholic Educational Association of the United States of America.

Codina, G (2000). The modus Parisiensis. *The Jesuit ratio studiorum: 400th anniversary perspectives.* New York: Fordham University Press.

Coleman, G. How the spiritual exercises inform the ministry of teaching. loyola.jesuit.org.au/cje/howthespiritual.html (site accessed 12/03/03).

Creighton University Bulletin. (2001). Holy university mission statement. Holy University Publications.

Creighton University Home Page. www.creighton.edu/ (site accessed 2/24/04).
Crowley, P (2002). The Jesuit university and the search for transcendence. *Conversations*, 22, 10-15.
Day, D & Scroope, M (2002). Ignatian ministry: From foundational insights to contemporary praxis. loyola.jesuit.org.au/opif/igmin.html (site accessed 12/03/02).
Downey, M (1991). Current trends understanding Christian spirituality: Dress rehearsal for a method. *Spirituality Today*, 43, 271-280. www.spiritualitytoday.org/spi2day/91433downey.html (site accessed 10/01/02).
Duminuco, V (2000). A new *Ratio* for a new millennium. *The Jesuit Ratio studiorum: 400th*. V Duminuco (ed.). New York: Fordham University Press.
Ellis, D (1980). Whatever happened to the spiritual dimension? *The Canadian Nurse*, 76, 42-43.
Emblen, J (1992). Religion and spirituality defined according to current use in nursing literature. *Journal of Professional Nursing*, 8, 41-47.
Feeney, J, Gilman, O & Parker, J (1997). Hiring faculty for mission: A case study of a department's search. *Conversations*, 12, 20-23.
Graves, F (1926). *A student's history of education*. New York: The Macmillan Company.
Harvanek, R (1989). *The Jesuit vision of a university*. Chicago: Loyola University.
Heft, J (1999). Have Catholic colleges reached an impasse? *The Chronicle of Higher Education*. www.chronicle.com (site accessed 7/31/02).
Holy Cross College. Jesuit educational traditions. www.holycross.edu/departments/jesuit/jesedtrad.html (site accessed 12/04/02).
International Center for Jesuit Education. (2002). *Ignatian pedagogy—a practical approach*. www.staloysius.nsw.edu.au/Jesuits/forward.htm
Johnson, E (1997). Misconceptions about the early land-grant colleges. *The history of higher education* (2nd ed). L Goodchild & H Wechsler (eds.). Needham Heights, MA: Simon & Schuster Custom Publishing.
Jones, A. Colleges & universities: Preserving mission and ministry at college. *NCR Online*. www.natcath.com/NCR_Online/archives/102502/102502u.thm (site accessed 11/26/02).
Kolvenbach, PH (1989). Themes of Jesuit Higher Education. (Key ideas contained in two addresses by the Superior General of the Society of Jesus delivered June 7, 1989, at Georgetown University and Georgetown Prep, summarized and edited by John J. Callahan, SJ.) www.creighton.edu/Heartland3/r-themes.html (site accessed 10/24/02).

———. (2000). The service of faith and the promotion of justice in American Jesuit higher education. http://www.sjweb.info/documents/doc_show.cfm?PubTextId=2014 (site accessed on 7-14-04).

———. (2001). The Jesuit university in the light of the Ignatian charism. Address of Fr. Peter-Hans Kolvenbach, Superior General of the Society of Jesus to the International Meeting of Jesuit Higher Education Rome (Monte Cucco). http://www.sjweb.info/documents/doc_show.cfm?PubTextId=1607 (site accessed 7-14-04).

Lannon, T (2001). The role of presidents promoting Catholic identity at Jesuit universities. *Conversations,* 20, 31-38.

Larson, D, Sawyers, JP & McCullough ME (1997). *Scientific research on spirituality and health: A consensus report.* Rockville MD: National Institute for Healthcare Research.

Maher, M, Shore, P & Parker, K (1999). From 1599-1999: Celebrating the *Ratio studiorum* at Saint Louis University. *Conversations,* 16, 47-51.

Matthews, R, Platt, D (1992). *The western humanities* (3rd ed). Mountain View CA: Mayfield Publishing Company.

McBrien, R (2001). *Lives of the saints.* San Francisco: Harper Collins Publishers.

McMurtrie, B (1999). How Catholic should Catholic colleges be? *The Chronicle of Higher Education.* (September 17). www.chronicle.com (site accessed 8/02/02).

Modras, R (2000). Rooted in the Renaissance: The Jesuit mission at Saint Louis University. *Conversations,* 18. 25-31.

Morrison, M (1995). *Creighton identity: We are university. We are Jesuit. We are Catholic.* Creighton University Publications.

Moser, M (2002). A warm heart and a clear eye: *Ex corde ecclesiae* and the university. *Conversations,* 22, 19-23.

National Conference of Catholic Bishops. (2000). *The application of Ex corde ecclesiae for the United States.* United States Catholic Conference, Inc., Washington D.C.

O'Brien, D (1994). Conversation on Jesuit (and Catholic?) higher education: Jesuit si, Catholic...not so sure. *Conversations,* 6, 4-13.

———. (1994). *From the heart of the American church: Catholic higher education and American culture.* Maryknoll, NY: Orbis Books.

O'Hare, J (1999). *Ex corde eccleasiae* - the history of the issue. www.accunet.org/ece/history.asp (site accessed 11/26/02).

O'Malley, J (1999). Introduction: *Ratio studiorum*—Jesuit education, 1548-1773. www.accunet.org/display.asp?category=14&page=2 (site accessed 7/22/04).

———. (2000). How the first Jesuits became involved in education, *The Jesuit ratio studiorum: 400th anniversary perspectives.* V Duminuco. (ed.). New York: Fordham University Press.

Padberg, J (1999) Companions in the mission of Christ. Ignatian Spirituality Conference. www.slu.edu/conferences/isc/padberg.html (site accessed 10/03/02).

Passon, R (1997). Hiring for mission: An overview. *Conversations,* 12, 5-13.

Pope John Paul II (1990). *Ex corde ecclesiae.* www.cin.org/jp2/excorde.html (site accessed 3/12/01).

Puhl, L (1951). *The spiritual exercises of St. Ignatius.* Chicago: Loyola Press.

Schlegel J (2000). Embracing the future together. President's inaugural response. www.creighton.edu/president/speeces/Inaugural.html (site accessed 7/24/04).

Sharkey, P. Ignatian pedagogical paradigm. loyola.jesuit.org.au/opif/ipp.html (site accessed 12/03/02).

The Loyola Institute. *Ignatius, the first Jesuit schools and the Ratio studiorum.* loyola.jesuit.org.au/cje/ratio.html (site accessed 12/03/02).

Tisdell, E (2001). Spirituality in adult and higher education. ERIC Digest: ED459370. ericir.syr.edu/plweb-cgi/obtain.pl (site accessed 9/24/02).

Tylenda, JN (2001). *A pilgrim's journey: The autobiography of St. Ignatius.* San Francisco: Ignatius Press.

Veysey, R (1965). *The emergence of the American university.* Chicago: University of Chicago Press.

Walsh, M (1991). *Butler's lives of the saints.* Australia: Harper Collins Publishers.

Wilson, C (2001). Implementation of *Ex corde ecclesiae* in the United States: The civil law implications for American Catholic colleges. Presented at the Annual Meeting of the Association of Catholic Colleges & Universities. www.accunet.org/display.asp?category=14&page=4 (site accessed 11/26/02).

3. Peter-Hans Kolvenbach, SJ

The Service of Faith and the Promotion of Justice in American Jesuit Higher Education

EDITORIAL NOTE: An Address on Commitment to Justice in Jesuit Higher Education, Santa Clara University, October 6, 2000[1]

I. Introduction

This conference on the commitment to justice in American Jesuit higher education comes at an important moment in the rich history of the 28 colleges and universities represented here this evening. We also join Santa Clara University in celebrating the 150th anniversary of its founding.

Just as significant as this moment in history, is our location. Santa Clara Valley, named after the mission at the heart of this campus, is known worldwide as "Silicon Valley," the home of the microchip. Surely when Father Nobili, the founder of this university, saw the dilapidated church and compound of the former Franciscan mission, he could never have imagined this valley as the center of a global technological revolution.

This juxtaposition of mission and microchip is emblematic of all the Jesuit schools. Originally founded to serve the educational and religious needs of poor immigrant populations, they have become highly sophisticated institutions of learning in the midst of global wealth, power and culture. The turn of the millennium finds them in all their diversity: they are larger, better equipped, more complex and professional than ever before and also more concerned about their Catholic Jesuit identity.

In the history of American Jesuit higher education, there is much to be grateful for, first to God and the church and surely to the many faculty, students, administrators and benefactors who have made it what it is today. But this conference brings you together from across the United States with guests from Jesuit universities elsewhere, not to congratulate one another but for a strategic purpose. On behalf of the complex, professional and pluralistic institutions you represent, you are here to face a question as difficult as it is central: how can the Jesuit colleges and universities in the United States express faith-filled concern for justice in what they are as Christian academies of higher learning, in what their faculty do and in what their students become?

As a contribution to your response, I would like to (1) reflect with you on what faith and justice has meant for Jesuits since 1975; (2) consider some concrete circumstances of today; (3) suggest what justice rooted in faith could mean in American Jesuit higher education; and (4) conclude with an agenda for the first decade of the years 2000.

II. The Jesuit Commitment to Faith and Justice—New in 1975

I begin by recalling another anniversary that this conference commemorates. Twenty-five years ago, ten years after the closing of the Second Vatican Council, Jesuit delegates from around the world gathered at the 32nd General Congregation (GC), to consider how the Society of Jesus was responding to the deep transformation of all church life that was called for and launched by Vatican II.

After much prayer and deliberation, the Congregation slowly realized that the entire Society of Jesus in all its many works was being invited by the Spirit of God to set out on a new direction. The overriding purpose of the Society of Jesus, namely "the service of faith," must also include "the promotion of justice." This new direction was not confined to those already working with the poor and marginalized in what was called "the social apostolate." Rather, this commitment was to be "a concern of our whole life and a dimension of all our apostolic endeavors"(General Congregation 32, 1974-5, D 4, n. 47).

Service of Faith & Promotion of Justice in Jesuit Higher Education 51

So central to the mission of the entire Society was this union of faith and justice that it was to become the "integrating factor" of all the Society's works (General Congregation 32, 1974-5, D 2, n. 9) and in this light "great attention" was to be paid in evaluating every work, including educational institutions.[2]

I myself attended GC 32, representing the province of the Near East where, for centuries, the apostolic activity of the Jesuits has concentrated on education in a famous university and some outstanding high schools. Of course some Jesuits worked in very poor villages, refugee camps or prisons and some fought for the rights of workers, immigrants and foreigners; but this was not always considered authentic, mainstream Jesuit work. In Beirut we were well aware that our medical school, staffed by very holy Jesuits, was producing, at least at that time, some of the most corrupt citizens in the city, but this was taken for granted. The social mood of the explosive Near East did not favor a struggle against sinful, unjust structures. The liberation of Palestine was the most important social issue. The Christian churches had committed themselves to many works of charity, but involvement in the promotion of justice would have tainted them by association with leftist movements and political turmoil.

The situation I describe in the Near East was not exceptional in the worldwide Society at that time. I was not the only delegate who was ignorant of matters pertaining to justice and injustice. The 1971 World Synod of Catholic Bishops had prophetically declared, "Action on behalf of justice and participation in the transformation of the world fully appear to us as a constitutive dimension of the preaching of the gospel or, in other words, of the church's mission for the redemption of the human race and its liberation from every oppressive situation" (World Synod of Catholic Bishops, 1971), but few of us knew what this meant in our concrete circumstances.

Earlier, in 1966, Father Arrupe had pointed out to the Latin American provincials how the socioeconomic situation throughout the continent contradicted the gospel and "from this situation rises the moral obligation of the Society to rethink all its ministries and every form of its apostolates to see if they really offer a response to the urgent priorities that justice and social equity call for"(Arrupe, 1996, p. 791). Many of us failed to see the relevance of his message to our situation. But please note that Father Arrupe did not ask for the suppression of the apostolate of education in favor of social activity. On the contrary, he affirmed that "even an apostolate like education—at all levels—which is so sincerely wanted by the Society and whose importance is clear to the entire world, in its concrete forms today must be the object of reflection in the light of the demands of the social problem"(Arrupe, 1996, p. 791).

Perhaps the incomprehension or reluctance of some of us delegates was one reason why GC 32 finally took a radical stand. With a passion both inspiring and disconcerting, the General Congregation coined the formula, "the service of faith and the promotion of justice" and used it adroitly to push every Jesuit work and every individual Jesuit to make a choice, providing little leeway for the fainthearted. Many inside and outside the Society were outraged by the "promotion of justice." As Father Arrupe rightly perceived, his Jesuits were collectively entering upon a more severe way of the cross that would surely entail misunderstandings and even opposition on the part of civil and ecclesiastical authorities, many good friends and some of our own members. Today, 25 years later, this option has become integral to our Jesuit identity, to the awareness of our mission and to our public image in both church and society (Kolvenbach, 2000).

The summary expression "the service of faith and the promotion of justice" has all the characteristics of a world-conquering slogan using a minimum of words to inspire a maximum of dynamic vision but at the risk of ambiguity. Let us examine, first the service of faith, then the promotion of justice.

A. The Service of Faith

From our origins in 1540 the Society has been officially and solemnly charged with "the defense and the propagation of the faith." In 1975, the Congregation reaffirmed that for us Jesuits the defense and propagation of the faith is a matter of "to be or not to be," even if the words themselves can change. Faithful to the Vatican Council, the Congregation wanted our preaching and teaching not to proselytize, not to impose our religion on others, but rather to propose Jesus and his message of God's Kingdom in a spirit of love to everyone.

Just as the Vatican had abandoned the name *"propaganda fidei,"* GC 32 passed from propagation to *service* of faith. In Decree 4, the Congregation did use the expression "the proclamation of faith," which I prefer.[3] In the context of centuries of Jesuit spirituality, however, "the service of faith" cannot mean anything other than to bring the counter-cultural gift of Christ to our world (General Congregation 32, 1974-5, D 26, n. 5). But why "the service of faith?" The Congregation itself answers this question by using the Greek expression *"diakonia fidei."*[4] It refers to Christ the suffering servant carrying out his *"diakonia"* in total service to his Father by laying down his life for the salvation of all. Thus, for a Jesuit, "Not just any response to the needs of the men and women of today will do. The initiative must come from the Lord laboring in events and people here and now. God invites us to follow Christ in his labors, on his terms and in his way" (General Congregation 34, 1995, D 26, n. 8).

I do not think we delegates at the 32nd Congregation were aware of the theological and ethical dimensions of Christ's mission of service. Greater attention to the *"diakonia fidei"* may have prevented some of the misunderstandings provoked by the phrase "the promotion of justice."

B. The Promotion of Justice

This expression is difficult to translate in many languages. We delegates were familiar with sales promotions in a department store or the promotion of friends or enemies to a higher rank or position. We were not familiar with the promotion of justice. To be fair, let us remember that a General Congregation is not a scientific academy equipped to distinguish and to define, to clarify and to classify. In the face of radically new apostolic needs, it chose to inspire, to teach and even to prophesy. In its desire to be more incisive in the promotion of justice, the Congregation avoided traditional words like charity, mercy—or love—unfashionable words in 1975. Neither philanthropy nor even development would do. The Congregation instead used the word "promotion" with its connotation of a well-planned strategy to make the world just.

Since Saint Ignatius wanted love to be expressed not only in words but also in deeds, the Congregation committed the Society to the promotion of justice as a concrete, radical, but proportionate, response to an unjustly suffering world. Fostering the virtue of justice in people was not enough. Only a substantive justice can bring about the kinds of structural and attitudinal changes that are needed to uproot those sinful oppressive injustices that are a scandal against humanity and God.

This sort of justice requires an action-oriented commitment to the poor with a courageous personal option. In some ears the relatively mild expression, "promotion of justice," echoed revolutionary, subversive and even violent language. For example, the American State Department recently accused some Colombian Jesuits of being Marxist-inspired founders of a guerilla organization. When challenged the government apologized for this mistake, which shows that some message did get through.

Just as in "*diakonia fidei*" the term faith is not specified, so in the "promotion of justice," the term justice also remains ambiguous. The 32nd Congregation would not have voted for Decree 4 if, on the one hand, socioeconomic justice had been excluded or if, on the other hand, the justice of the gospel had not been included. A stand in favor of social justice that was almost ideological and simultaneously a strong option for "that justice of the Gospel that embodies God's love and saving mercy" (General Congregation 33, 1983, D 1, n. 32) were both indispensable. Refusing to clarify the relationship between the two, GC 32 maintained its radicality by simply juxtaposing "*diakonia fidei*" and "promotion of justice."

In other decrees of the same Congregation, when the two dimensions of the one mission of the Society were placed together, some delegates sought to achieve a more integrated expression by proposing amendments such as the service of faith *through* or *in* the promotion of justice. Such expressions might better render the 1971 Synod's identification of "action on behalf of justice and participation in the transformation of the world [as] a constitutive dimension of the preaching of the gospel" (World Synod of Catholic Bishops, 1971).

But one can understand the Congregation's fear that too neat or integrated an approach might weaken the prophetic appeal and water down the radical change in our mission.

In retrospect, this simple juxtaposition sometimes led to an "incomplete, slanted and unbalanced reading" of Decree 4 (Arrupe, 1981), unilaterally emphasizing "one aspect of this mission to the detriment of the other" (General Congregation of the Society of Jesus 33, 1983), treating faith and justice as alternative or even rival tracks of ministry. "Dogmatism or ideology sometimes led us to treat each other more as adversaries than as companions. The promotion of justice has sometimes been separated from its wellspring of faith" (General Congregation of the Society of Jesus 34, 1995).

On the one side, the faith dimension was too often presumed and left implicit, as if our identity as Jesuits were enough. Some rushed headlong towards the promotion of justice without much analysis or reflection and with only occasional reference to the justice of the gospel. They seemed to consign the service of faith to a dying past.

Those on the other side clung to a certain style of faith and church. They gave the impression that God's grace had to do only with the next life and that divine reconciliation entailed no practical obligation to set things right here on earth.

In this frank assessment I have used, not so much my own words but rather those of subsequent Congregations, so as to share with you the whole Society's remorse for whatever distortions or excesses occurred and to demonstrate how, over the last 25 years, the Lord has patiently been teaching us to serve the faith that does justice in a more integral way.

C. The Ministry of Education

In the midst of radical statements and unilateral interpretations associated with Decree 4, many raised doubts about our maintaining large educational institutions. They insinuated, if they did not insist, that direct social work among the poor and involvement with their movements should take priority. Today, however, the value of the educational apostolate is generally recognized, being the sector occupying the most Jesuit manpower and resources, but only on condition that it transform its goals, contents and methods.

Even before GC 32, Father Arrupe had already fleshed out the meaning of "*diakonia fidei*" for educational ministries when he told the 1973 International Congress of Jesuit Alumni of Europe: "Today our prime educational objective must be to form men for others; men who will live not for themselves but for God and his Christ - for the God-man who lived and died for all the world; men who cannot even conceive of love of God that does not include love for the least of their neighbors; men completely convinced that love of God that does not issue in justice for men is a farce" (Arrupe, 1983). My predecessor's address was not well received by many alumni at the Valencia meeting, but the expression "men and women for others" really helped the educational institutions of the Society to ask serious questions that led to their transformation (Jesuit Secondary Education Association, 1987).

Father Ignacio Ellacuría, in his 1982 convocation address here at Santa Clara University, eloquently expressed his conviction in favor of the promotion of justice in the educational apostolate: "A Christian university must take into account the gospel preference for the poor. This does not mean that only the poor study at the university; it does not mean that the university should abdicate its mission of academic excellence - excellence needed in order to solve complex social problems. It does mean that the university should be present intellectually where it is needed: to provide science for those who have no science; to provide skills for the unskilled; to be a voice for those who do not possess the academic qualifications to promote and legitimate their rights" (Ellacuría, 1982).

In these two statements, we discover the same concern to go beyond a disincarnate spiritualism or a secular social activism, so as to renew the educational apostolate in word and in action at the service of the church in a world of unbelief and of injustice. We should be very grateful for all that has been achieved in this apostolate, both faithful to the characteristics of 400 years of Ignatian education and open to the changing signs of the times. Today, one or two generations after Decree 4, we face a world that has an even greater need for the faith that does justice.

III. A "Composition" of Our Time and Place

The 25-year history we lived through and have briefly surveyed, brings us to the present. Ignatius of Loyola begins many meditations in his *Spiritual Exercises* with "a composition of place," an exercise of the imagination to situate prayerful contemplation in concrete human circumstances. Since this world is the arena of God's presence and activity, Ignatius believes that we can find God if we approach the world with generous faith and a discerning spirit.

Meeting in Silicon Valley brings to mind, not only the intersection of the mission and the microchip but also the dynamism and even dominance that are characteristics of the United States at this time. Enormous talent and unprecedented prosperity are concentrated in this country, which spawns sixty-four new millionaires every day. This is the headquarters of the new economy that reaches around the globe and is transforming the basic fabric of business, work and communications. Thousands of immigrants arrive from everywhere: entrepreneurs from Europe, high-tech professionals from South Asia who staff the service industries as well as workers from Latin America and Southeast Asia who do the physical labor—thus, a remarkable ethnic, cultural and class diversity.

At the same time the United States struggles with new social divisions aggravated by "the digital divide" between those with access to the world of technology and those left out. This rift, with its causes in class, racial and economic differences, has its root cause in chronic discrepancies in the quality of education. Here in Silicon Valley, for example, some of the world's premier research universities flourish alongside struggling public schools where Afro-American and immigrant students drop out in droves. Nationwide, one child in every six is condemned to ignorance and poverty.

This valley, this nation and the whole world look very different from the way they looked 25 years ago. With the collapse of communism and the end of the Cold War, national and even international politics have been eclipsed by a resurgent capitalism that faces no ideological rival. The European Union slowly pulls the continent's age-old rivals together into a community but also a fortress. The former "Second World" struggles to repair the human and environmental damage left behind by so-called socialist regimes. Industries are relocating to poorer nations, not to distribute wealth and opportunity, but to exploit the relative advantage of low wages and lax environmental regulations. Many countries become yet poorer, especially where corruption and exploitation prevail over civil society and where violent conflict keeps erupting.

This composition of our time and place embraces six billion people with their faces young and old, some being born and others dying, some white and many brown and yellow and black.[5] Each one a unique individual, they all aspire to live life, to use their talents, to support their families and care for their children and elders, to enjoy peace and security and to make tomorrow better.

Thanks to science and technology, human society is able to solve problems such as feeding the hungry, sheltering the homeless or developing more just conditions of life, but remains stubbornly unable to accomplish this. How can a booming economy, the most prosperous and global ever, still leave over half of humanity in poverty? GC 32 makes its own sober analysis and moral assessment:

> We can no longer pretend that the inequalities and injustices of our world must be borne as part of the inevitable order of things. It is now quite apparent that they are the result of what man himself, man in his selfishness, has done. . . . Despite the opportunities offered by an ever more serviceable technology, we are simply not willing to pay the price of a more just and more humane society (General Congregation of the Society of Jesus 32, 1974-5, D 4, nn. 27, 20).

Injustice is rooted in a spiritual problem and its solution requires a spiritual conversion of each one's heart and a cultural conversion of our global society so that humankind, with all the powerful means at its disposal, might exercise the will to change the sinful structures afflicting our world. The yearly *Human Development Report* of the United Nations is a haunting challenge to look critically at basic conditions of life in the United States and the 175 other nations that share our one planet (United Nations Development Program, 1990). Such is the world in all its complexity, with great global promises and countless tragic betrayals. Such is the world in which Jesuit institutions of higher education are called to serve faith and promote justice.

IV. American Jesuit Higher Education for Faith and Justice

Within the complex time and place we are in and in the light of the recent General Congregations, I want to spell out several *ideal characteristics*, as manifest in three complementary dimensions of Jesuit higher education: in whom our students become; in what our faculty do; and in how our universities proceed. When I speak of ideals, some are easy to meet, others remain persistently challenging, but together they serve to orient our schools and, in the long run, to identify them. At the same time, the US provincials have recently established an important Higher Education Committee to propose *criteria* on the staffing, leadership and Jesuit sponsorship of our colleges and universities.[6] May these criteria help to implement the ideal characteristics we now meditate on together.

A. Formation and Learning

Today's predominant ideology reduces the human world to a global jungle whose primordial law is the survival of the fittest. Students who subscribe to this view want to be equipped with well-honed professional and technical skills in order to compete in the market and secure one of the relatively scarce fulfilling and lucrative jobs available. This is the success that many students (and parents!) expect.

All American universities, ours included, are under tremendous pressure to opt entirely for success in this sense. But what our students want—and deserve—includes but transcends this "worldly success" based on marketable skills. *The real measure of our Jesuit universities lies in whom our students become.*

For four hundred and fifty years, Jesuit education has sought to educate "the whole person" intellectually and professionally, psychologically, morally and spiritually. But in the emerging global reality, with its great possibilities and deep contradictions, the whole person is different from the whole person of the Counter-Reformation, the Industrial Revolution or the 20th century. Tomorrow's "whole person" cannot be whole without an educated awareness of society and culture with which to contribute socially—generously—in the real world. Tomorrow's whole person must have, in brief, a *well-educated solidarity*.

We must therefore raise our Jesuit educational standard to "educate the whole person of solidarity for the real world." Solidarity is learned through "contact" rather than through "concepts," as the Holy Father said recently at an Italian university conference (John Paul II, 1984). When the heart is touched by direct experience, the mind may be challenged to change. Personal involvement with innocent suffering, with the injustice others suffer is the catalyst for solidarity that then gives rise to intellectual inquiry and moral reflection.

Students, in the course of their formation, must let the gritty reality of this world into their lives, so they can learn to feel it, think about it critically, respond to its suffering and engage it constructively. They should learn to perceive, think, judge, choose and act for the rights of others, especially the disadvantaged and the oppressed. Campus ministry does much to foment such intelligent, responsible and active compassion, compassion that deserves the name solidarity.

Our universities also boast a splendid variety of in-service programs, outreach programs, insertion programs, off-campus contacts and hands-on courses. These should not be too optional or peripheral, but at the core of every Jesuit university's program of studies.

Our students are involved in every sort of social action—tutoring dropouts, demonstrating in Seattle, serving in soup kitchens, promoting pro-life, protesting against the School of the Americas—and we are proud of them for it. But the measure of Jesuit universities is not what our students do but whom they become and the adult Christian responsibility they will exercise in future towards their neighbor and their world. For now, the activities they engage in, even with much good effect, are for their formation. This does not make the university a training camp for social activists. Rather, the students need close involvement with the poor and the marginal now, in order to learn about reality and become adults of solidarity in the future.

B. Research and Teaching

If the measure and purpose of our universities lie in what the students become, then the faculty are at the heart of our universities. Their mission is tirelessly to seek the truth and to form each student into a whole person of solidarity who will take responsibility for the real world. What do they need in order to fulfil this essential vocation?

The faculty's "research, which must be rationally rigorous, firmly rooted in faith and open to dialogue with all people of good will" (John Paul II, 2000), not only obeys the canons of each discipline but ultimately embraces human reality in order to help make the world a more fitting place for six billion of us to inhabit. I want to affirm that university knowledge is valuable for its own sake and at the same time is knowledge that must ask itself, "For whom? For what?" (General Congregation of the Society of Jesus 34, 1995).

Usually we speak of professors in the plural, but what is at stake is more than the sum of so many individual commitments and efforts. It is a sustained interdisciplinary dialogue of research and reflection, a continuous pooling of expertise. The purpose is to assimilate experiences and insights according to their different disciplines in "a vision of knowledge which, well aware of its limitations, is not satisfied with fragments but tries to integrate them into a true and wise synthesis" (John Paul II, 2000) about the real world. Unfortunately many faculty still feel academically, humanly and I would say spiritually, unprepared for such an exchange.

In some disciplines such as the life sciences, the social sciences, law, business or medicine, the connections with "our time and place" may seem more obvious. These professors apply their disciplinary specialties to issues of justice and injustice in their research and teaching about health care, legal aid, public policy and international relations. But every field or branch of knowledge has values to defend, with repercussions on the ethical level. Every discipline, beyond its necessary specialization, must engage with human society, human life and the environment in appropriate ways, cultivating moral concern about how people ought to live together.

All professors, in spite of the cliché of the ivory tower, are in contact with the world. But no point of view is ever neutral or value-free. By preference, by option, our Jesuit point of view is that of the poor. So our professors' commitment to faith and justice entails a most significant shift in viewpoint and choice of values. Adopting the point of view of those who suffer injustice, our professors seek the truth and share their search and its results with our students. A legitimate question, even if it does not sound academic, is for each professor to ask, "When researching and teaching, where and with whom is my heart?" To expect our professors to make such an explicit option and speak about it is obviously not easy; it entails risks. But I do believe that this is what Jesuit educators have publicly stated, in church and in society, to be our defining commitment.

To make sure that the real concerns of the poor find their place in research, faculty members need an organic collaboration with those in the church and in society who work among and for the poor and actively seek justice. They should be involved together in all aspects: presence among the poor, designing the research, gathering the data, thinking through problems, planning and action, doing evaluation and theological reflection. In each Jesuit province where our universities are found, the faculty's privileged working relationships should be with projects of the Jesuit social apostolate - on issues such as poverty and exclusion, housing, AIDS, ecology and Third World debt - and with the Jesuit Refugee Service helping refugees and forcibly displaced people.

Just as the students need the poor in order to learn, so the professors need partnerships with the social apostolate in order to research and teach and form. Such partnerships do not turn Jesuit universities into branch plants of social ministries or agencies of social change, as certain rhetoric of the past may have led some to fear, but are a verifiable pledge of the faculty's option, and they really help, as the colloquial expression goes, "to keep your feet to the fire!"

If the professors choose viewpoints incompatible with the justice of the gospel and consider researching, teaching and learning to be separable from moral responsibility for their social repercussions, they are sending a message to their students. They are telling them that they can pursue their careers and self-interest without reference to anyone other than themselves.

By contrast, when faculty do take up interdisciplinary dialogue and socially-engaged research in partnership with social ministries, they are exemplifying and modeling knowledge which is service and the students learn by imitating them as "masters of life and of moral commitment" (John Paul II, 1984), as the Holy Father said.

C. Our Way of Proceeding

If the measure of our universities is who the students become and if the faculty are the heart of it all, then what is there left to say? It is perhaps the third topic, the character of our universities - how they proceed internally and how they impact on society - that is the most difficult.

We have already dwelt on the importance of formation and learning, of research and teaching. The social action that the students undertake and the socially-relevant work that the professors do, are vitally important and necessary, but these do not add up to the full character of a Jesuit university. They neither exhaust its faith-justice commitment nor really fulfill its responsibilities to society.

What, then, constitutes this ideal character? And what contributes to the public's perception of it? In the case of a Jesuit university, this character must surely be the mission that is defined by GC 32 and reaffirmed by GC 34: the *diakonia fidei* and the promotion of justice, as the characteristic Jesuit university way of proceeding and of serving socially. In the words of GC 34, a Jesuit university must be faithful to both the noun "university" and to the adjective "Jesuit." To be a university requires dedication "to research, teaching and the various forms of service that correspond to its cultural mission." To be Jesuit "requires that the university act in harmony with the demands of the service of faith and promotion of justice found in Decree 4 of GC 32" (D 17, nn. 6,7).

The first way, historically, that our universities began living out their faith-justice commitment was through their admissions policies, affirmative action for minorities and scholarships for disadvantaged students;[7] and these continue to be effective means. An even more telling expression of the Jesuit university's nature is found in policies concerning hiring and tenure. As a *university* it is necessary to respect the established academic, professional and labor norms, but as *Jesuit* it is essential to go beyond them and find ways of attracting, hiring and promoting those who actively share the mission.

I believe that we have made considerable and laudable *Jesuit* efforts to go deeper and further: we have brought our Ignatian spirituality, our reflective capacities, some of our international resources, to bear. Good results are evident, for example, in the decree *Jesuits and University Life* of the last General Congregation and in this very Conference on "Commitment to Justice in Jesuit Higher Education"; and good results are hoped for from the Higher Education Committee working on Jesuit criteria.

Paraphrasing Ignacio Ellacuría, it is the nature of every university to be a social force and it is the calling of a Jesuit university to take conscious responsibility for being such a force for faith and justice. Every Jesuit academy of higher learning is called to live in a social reality (as we saw in the "composition" of our time and place) and to live for that social reality, to shed university intelligence upon it and to use university influence to transform it (Ellacuría, 1982). Thus Jesuit universities have stronger and different reasons than many other academic and research institutions for addressing the actual world as it unjustly exists and for helping to reshape it in the light of the gospel.

V. In Conclusion—an Agenda

The 25th anniversary of GC 32 is a motive for great thanksgiving.

We give thanks for our Jesuit university awareness of the world in its entirety and in its ultimate depth, created yet abused, sinful yet redeemed. We take up our Jesuit university responsibility for human society that is so scandalously unjust, so complex to understand and so hard to change. With the help of others and especially the poor, we want to play our role as students, as teachers and researchers and as Jesuit universities in society. As Jesuit higher education, we embrace new ways of learning and being formed in the pursuit of adult solidarity; new methods of researching and teaching in an academic community of dialogue; and a new university way of practicing faith-justice in society.

As we assume our Jesuit university characteristics in the new century, we do so with seriousness and hope. For this very mission has produced martyrs who prove that "an institution of higher learning and research can become an instrument of justice in the name of the gospel" (Kolvenbach, 1990). But implementing Decree 4 is not something a Jesuit university accomplishes once and for all. It is rather an ideal to keep taking up and working at, a cluster of characteristics to keep exploring and implementing, a conversion to keep praying for.

In *Ex Corde Ecclesiae,* Pope John Paul II charges Catholic universities with a challenging agenda for teaching, research and service: "The dignity of human life, the promotion of justice for all, the quality of personal and family life, the protection of nature, the search for peace and political stability, a more just sharing in the world's resources and a new economic and political order that will better serve the human community at a national and international level" (Pope John Paul II, 1990). These are both high ideals and concrete tasks. I encourage our Jesuit colleges and universities to take them up with critical understanding and deep conviction, with buoyant faith and much hope in the early years of the new century.

The beautiful words of the GC show us a long path to follow: "The way to faith and the way to justice are inseparable ways. It is up this undivided road, this steep road, that the pilgrim Church" - the Society of Jesus, the Jesuit college and university— "must travel and toil. Faith and justice are undivided in the Gospel which teaches that 'faith makes its power felt through love' (Galatians 5:6) They cannot therefore be divided in our purpose, our action, our life" (General Congregation of the Society of Jesus 32, 1974-5, D 2, n. 8). For the greater glory of God.

Thank you very much.

Notes

[1] Published previously in *Studies in the Spirituality of Jesuits* (2001). 31(1) 1-29.
http://www.scu.edu/news/releases.cfm/1000/kolvenbach_speech.html (site accessed 7/22/04).
[2] See GC 32, D.2, n. 9 and D.4, n. 76.
[3] "Since evangelisation is proclamation of that faith which is made operative in love of others (see Galatians 5:6; Ephesians 4:15), the promotion of justice is indispensable to it" (GC32, D. 4, n. 28).
[4] For example, GC32, D. 11, n. 13.
[5] See "Contemplation on the Incarnation," Ignatius of Loyola, *Spiritual exercises*, nos. 101-109.
[6] In February 2000, the Jesuit Conference established a five-man Committee on Higher Education to prepare recommendations regarding (1) sponsorship by the Society of US Jesuit colleges and universities; 2) assignment of personnel to these institutions; 3) selection of presidents (particularly non-Jesuit presidents) for these institutions.
[7] "For the poor [the universities] serve as major channels for social advancement" (GC34, D. 17, n. 2).

References

Arrupe, SJ P (1966). On the social apostolate in Latin America, December. *Acta Romana Societatis, Iesu, XIV.*

———. (1981). Rooted and grounded in love. *Acta Romana Societatis, Iesu, XVIII.*

———. (1983). Address to the European Jesuit Alumni Congress. Valencia, Spain, August 1973. In *Hombres para los demás*. Barcelona: Diafora.

Ellacuría, SJ, I (1982). The task of a Christian university. Convocation address at the University of Santa Clara, June 12. Una universidad para el pueblo. *Diakonía*. 6 (23).

General Congregation of the Society of Jesus 32 (1974-5).

General Congregation of the Society of Jesus 33 (1983).

General Congregation of the Society of Jesus 34 (1995).

Jesuit Secondary Education Association (1987). *The characteristics of Jesuit education*. Washington, DC: Jesuit Secondary Education Association.

John Paul II (2000). Address to the Catholic University of the Sacred Heart, Milan, Italy, May 5.

———. (1984). Address to the Faculty of Medicine, Catholic University of the Sacred Heart, Milan, Italy, June 26.

———. (1990) *Ex corde eccleasiae.* www.cin.org/jp2/excorde.html (site accessed 7/22/04).

Kolvenbach, SJ, PH (2000). On the social apostolate. January. (1990). Address to the congregation of provincials. *Acta Romana Societatis, Iesu.*

World Synod of Catholic Bishops (1971). Justice in the world. In DJ O'Brien & A Shannon (eds.). *Catholic social thought: The documentary heritage.* Maryknoll, NY: Orbis Books.

United Nations Development Program (1990). *Human development report. 1990-present.* Government Publications UN2 DE -H72. http://www.undp.org/hdro (site accessed 7/22/04).

4. Thomas Massaro, SJ

A Preferential Option for the Poor: Historical & Theological Foundations

> The option for the poor, with all of the pastoral and theological consequences of that option, is one of the most important contributions to the life of the church universal to have emerged from the theology of liberation and the church on our continent. As we have observed, that option has its roots in biblical revelation and the history of the church. Still, today it presents particular, novel characteristics.
>
> Gustavo Gutiérrez
> *Option for the Poor*

I. Introduction

The "preferential option for the poor" has become a point of controversy and frequent misunderstanding in recent decades. Since the initial coining of this phrase in Latin America in the 1970s as an attempt to describe God's special relationship with disadvantaged people, and the resulting moral obligations that fall upon the privileged in our age, this concept has been championed as well as vilified by numerous observers, both inside and outside the Catholic church.

This essay seeks to provide an overview of the theological notion of preferential option for the poor for non-theologians. We explore just enough of the historical and biblical background of this contested concept to supply a point of entry for health care ethicists and policy analysts to appreciate how it might be applied to their fields of study and concern. After surveying the scriptural, theological and historical roots of the concept, we move beyond abstractions and generalizations to a concrete example of how the preferential option for the poor has inspired one particular group of people (the Jesuits of Latin America) to reshape a long-standing commitment to institutions that affect the prospects of millions.

The option for the poor, above all, is about social engagement. It calls the non-poor who accept it to undertake concrete actions that embody solidarity and social concern for the least advantaged. The key insight starts as an epistemological one (seeing reality through the eyes of the poor and marginalized) and proceeds to issue forth in commitments to social reform to address the causes and effects of poverty. Some of the appropriate responses might take the form of individual and episodic actions of charity and compassion such as the giving of alms or voluntary service. Other approaches to social reform inspired by a preferential option for the poor require collective and more systematic responses, such as advocating for structural changes in key social systems: law, medicine, politics and the economy. Precisely because these social systems are invariably controlled by elite members of society, an option for the poor on the part of the privileged emerges as essential for the prospect of social change.

II. The Turn toward Justice

In recent decades, these insights have guided the Catholic church around the world to supplement its previous "charity alone" approach with a "justice building upon charity" orientation. Church leaders and documents since the Second Vatican Council (1962-65) have increasingly emphasized the crucial importance of structural change in a world divided so sharply between rich and poor. *Gaudium et Spes*, a key Vatican II document addressing the role of the church in contemporary society, lamented how "luxury and misery rub shoulders" in a world "where an enormous mass of people still lack the absolute necessities of life" while others "live sumptuously or squander wealth" (Pope Paul VI, 1992, par 63). The severity of this contrast between wealth and abject poverty, both among and within nations, is an occasion for discomfort on the part of all people of conscience but surely constitutes a source of dire alarm particularly for people of the Christian faith. The gospel of Jesus Christ, that poor man who dedicated his ministry especially to the lowly and outcast people of his day, calls us to do all we can to rectify this situation. In an important document that reflects the deliberations of hundreds of bishops brought together from around the world to consider the task of achieving justice in our day, the 1971 World Synod of Catholic Bishops declared:

> Action on behalf of justice and participation in the transformation of the world fully appear to us as a constitutive dimension of the preaching of the Gospel, or, in other words, of the Church's mission for the redemption of the human race and its liberation from every oppressive situation (World Synod of Catholic Bishops, 1971, par. 6).

The pursuit of justice is incumbent upon all who claim to be living out the Gospel. The "good news" of the Christian proclamation must always be good news for the poor, who demand the special attention of the non-poor.

We should not be surprised that the two Vatican documents quoted above do not explicitly cite the phrase preferential option for the poor, for the term was not used in any official church document until 1979, when the Latin American bishops decided to feature it prominently. Meeting in Puebla, Mexico, they enshrined this phrase in the magisterial idiom by entitling an entire section of their conference's final document "The Preferential Option for the Poor" (Puebla Final Document, 1979, part 4, ch. 1). Both before and since, church history has witnessed a number of circumlocutions and alternative ways of making this same point about the obligation of the privileged to stand in solidarity with the oppressed and marginalized. Indeed, at the risk of anachronism, we might go so far as to interpret the entire tradition of modern Catholic social teaching, as well as the biblical and theological resources upon which it draws, as incarnating and expressing a preferential option for the poor[1]. Let us investigate this bold claim.

III. The Poor in the Scriptures

As mentioned in the opening paragraph above, a key to understanding the force of the preferential option for the poor is the recognition that our obligation to develop and express solidarity with the poor is grounded in the affirmation that the Christian God has already made a divine preferential option for the poor. A continuous strand in the biblical witness to God's self-revelation highlights how divine favor has been heaped time and again upon the poor, the lowly and the outcast. We discover this theme of surprising reversal from the very beginning of the biblical narrative. In chapter four of Genesis, God favors the gift of Abel, the younger son, over that of Cain, the elder (and presumably more privileged) offspring of Adam and Eve. God's choice of the lowborn is a recurring theme of the Hebrew Scriptures, as unlikely kings, patriarchs and prophets are frequently chosen to carry out the will of Yahweh.

This leitmotif of the "Great Reversal" works its way into the Christian Scriptures as well. We find a particularly dramatic display of this theme in the Virgin Mary's Magnificat (Luke 1: 46-55), a canticle featuring praise for a God who has "raised the lowly to high places." We also see it in such writings of St. Paul as I Corinthians 1: 26-9:

> You are among those called. Consider your situation. Not many of you are wise, as men account wisdom; not many are influential; and surely not many are wellborn. God chose those whom the world considers absurd to shame the wise; he singled out the weak of this world to shame the strong. He chose the world's lowborn and despised, those who count for nothing, to reduce to nothing those who were something; so that mankind could do no boasting before God.

Numerous other passages, especially from the synoptic gospels, could be cited to substantiate a divine option for the poor. Some are brief summaries of the teaching of Jesus, such as Mark 2: 17 ("People who are healthy do not need a doctor; sick people do. I have come to call sinners, not the self-righteous"). Others are longer pericopes and even fully developed parables (e.g., the Last Judgment in Matthew 25: 31-46, in which Jesus closely identifies himself with the poorest and neediest by saying: "As often as you did it for one of my least brothers, you did it for me"). But none makes the point of the unmerited character of God's love more poetically than the Beatitudes, alternate forms of which appear in Matthew 5: 2-12 and Luke 6: 20-26. Each version in its own distinctive way singles out the poor, weak, humble, meek, hungry and sorrowing as finding favor with God. Luke's version appears to be more satisfying to proponents of a preferential option for the poor. Luke follows his Beatitudes ("Blessed are the . . . ") with a series of condemnations ("But woe to you rich . . . ; you who are full . . . ; you who laugh now . . . "). Further, Luke's first Beatitude reserves the reign of God for "the poor" rather than for "the poor in spirit" as in Matthew's version, which is often interpreted as referring to some "interior reality" and thus not demanding any material reforms at all. It is thus easy to comprehend how Matthew's version has come to be charged with "spiritualizing away" the meaning of poverty, although it is rightly argued that even this version of the Beatitudes spells good news for the poor and potential discomfort for the rich who grow complacent about their moral obligations.

If indeed the poor are blessed by God, the next question that might occur to an observer is the ethical one: precisely what are we to do about it? The Christian Scriptures offer us a few hints, but not very complete or satisfying treatments of this problem. In the parable of Dives (the rich man) and Lazarus (the beggar) in Luke 16: 19-31, the reader is led to infer that the rich are somehow in need of repentance if they are to escape the fires of hell. Perhaps their complicity in an economic system that mal-distributes wealth constitutes the basis of their culpability, although this is not clear in any explicit way from the details Luke provides. Even less helpful are those passages in Acts of the Apostles (2:44-5 and 4: 32-7) that describe in stylized language the economic arrangements of the primitive community of Christians, including these:

The community of believers were of one heart and one mind. None of them ever claimed anything as his own; rather, everything was held in common. . . . Nor was there anyone needy among them, for all who owned property or houses sold them and donated the proceeds. They used to lay them at the feet of the apostles to be distributed to everyone according to his need (Acts 4: 32, 34-5).

The impracticality of these idealized conditions is gainsaid even within the text of Acts (see chapter five for the story of Ananias and Sapphira who were struck dead for failure to share the full proceeds of the sale of their property). Subsequent commentators have rightly remarked that it becomes impossible to help the poor in a reliable and ongoing way once you pauperize yourself, and that communal sharing of property seldom works well or for long on a large scale.

Perhaps because they were associated with an established nation rather than a small and scattered group like first-century Christianity, the Hebrew Scriptures provide more practical and programmatic guidelines for assisting the poor. Many books of the prophets (especially Amos and Jeremiah) scold Israel for failing to practice social justice in accordance with the covenant between the chosen people and God. That Yahweh included concern for the vulnerable in the original covenant with Israel is amply demonstrated in core passages of the Torah, particularly sections of the book of Deuteronomy. For example, Deuteronomy 10: 18-19 describes God as one "who executes justice for the orphan and the widow and befriends the alien, feeding and clothing him. So you too must befriend the alien, for you were once aliens yourselves in the land of Egypt." In Deuteronomy 15, we are instructed in the types of financial arrangements that will help the poor: lending freely to meet the needs of the poor ("I command you to open your hand to your poor and needy kinsman") coupled with the practice of periodic relaxation of debts (see also Leviticus 25 on the sabbatical and jubilee years). Deuteronomy 24 repeats these injunctions favoring the marginalized (particularly the triad of widows, orphans and aliens) and adds a stipulation that part of each harvest is to be left in the fields so that the poor of the land may gather what they need to sustain themselves (see also Leviticus 19: 9-10 and 23:22).

Even from this brief survey of Holy Scripture we may discern a basic pattern of faith-based reflection on the proper attitude regarding poverty. All those who claim a relationship with God are called to recognize a moral obligation to stand in solidarity with the poor. There is surely room for a variety of potential responses to the dire needs of the marginalized, as a variety of social theories and approaches to poverty (from "bootstraps capitalism" to "cradle-to-grave socialism"—each with its obvious drawbacks) might be employed by way of remedy and assistance. But even in the Scriptures, which are far from an economic blueprint, we see a profound but uneasy grappling with the need for systematic approaches to justice for the poor beyond just moralistic appeals for almsgiving.

If there are indeed a variety of possible ways of acting on the preferential option for the poor, then the question arises: are there any approaches to the plight of the poor that are strictly off limits and out of bounds for followers of the God of the scriptures? People of good will and biblical inspiration certainly do enjoy the freedom to develop a diverse variety of personal responses to the tug of conscience associated with an option for the poor. It seems, however, that at least two routes are completely inadequate. The first is utter apathy and noninvolvement. To recognize the image of the living God in our neighbors calls for some demonstrable response that draws us out of ourselves and contributes to making the struggle of the desperately poor at least somehow more tolerable and less inhumane. Ignoring the situation of the poorest is simply not acceptable, especially in a world where approximately 1.3 billion people live on less than one dollar per day (United Nations Development Program, 1999, p. 22). Those who conclude that "business as usual" is good enough should be challenged to take better notice of their surroundings and to ponder the full meaning of their religious beliefs and similar motivating principles.

The second approach that seems irreconcilable with the mainstream of the Judeo-Christian tradition of approaches to poverty is social Darwinism. This is a school of thought that ostensibly peaked in the nineteenth century, through the influence of such social theorists as Herbert Spencer, but that is still very much alive today. True social Darwinists claim not only that fierce competition is indeed, empirically speaking, "the way of the world," but also that, normatively speaking, it is right and fitting that competition should be the predominant ethos of the age, the major way that people relate to one another. Social progress, the argument runs, depends on the dynamics of competitive economic behavior that mirrors the biological behavior that drives the physical evolution of species. The elimination of those who cannot compete effectively ("the thinning of the herd") is a positive good, for it means that only the fittest survive. In a world of scarcity, charity for the unfit is a luxury we cannot afford. We hear arguments like these from some figures in the recently developed field of socio-biology and those who borrow its insights to apply them to various fields of human endeavor such as public policy.

This line of reasoning is so obviously at variance with the message of Christianity (indeed, of practically all other traditions of serious religious or philosophical reflection) that one can only wonder why it is taken seriously, either in its normative or empirical aspects. Yet social Darwinism remains as something of a "default position" that seems to insinuate itself as the ethos of arenas of intense competition such as economic markets and political and legal systems. It would be impossible to overstate the contrast between social Darwinism, where "the other" represents a constant threat, and the preferential option for the poor, where the needy other is perceived as being of infinite worth, indeed a locus of deep personal concern that might elicit substantial personal sacrifice.

The biblical roots of preferential option for the poor, as surveyed above, played out in rich ways in the history of Christianity, evident to the discerning eye long before anyone used the phrase explicitly. Enlightened church and civic leaders in many ages dedicated impressive efforts to improving the lives of the poorest members of society. In the Christian European society of the Middle Ages, through the milieu of Renaissance humanism, in the missionary movements of the early modern age and amidst the ferment and social challenges of the industrial era, men and women in the name of the gospel labored to improve the lot of the poor, struggling against the variety of forces that fostered the marginalization and exploitation of millions of the disadvantaged around the world. Some of these efforts have been heroic in nature, garnering broad and well-deserved recognition for the saints and philanthropists who undertook them. Others remained rather modest and ordinary, hardly capturing the attention of anyone, often not even the beneficiaries of the sacrifices themselves.

Naturally, efforts to enact a preferential option for the poor gained more explicit attention once the church began to develop an idiom for expressing the force of this moral obligation. This has largely unfolded within the tradition of modern Catholic social teaching, which began with the encyclical *Rerum Novarum* promulgated in 1891 by Pope Leo XIII. This document marked the first occasion when a leader of the Catholic church analyzed the new challenges of the industrial age and placed the church on the side of the workers in their struggle for decent working and living conditions. Subsequent popes, church councils and groupings of bishops have contributed to the articulation of precisely what it means to enact an option for the poor and why it is vitally necessary in our increasingly interdependent age. We have already seen a few insights from the Vatican II document *Gaudium et Spes*, specifically the way it decried the growing gap between the world's rich and poor. Elsewhere, in fact in its very opening sentences, this ground-breaking document identifies the church with the poor in this bold declaration:

> The joys and hopes, the griefs and anxieties of the men and women of this age, especially those who are poor or in any way afflicted, these too are the joys and hopes, the griefs and anxieties of the followers of Christ. Indeed, nothing genuinely human fails to raise an echo in their hearts (Pope Paul VI, 1979, par. 1).

This introduction to the document reflects the sentiments of Pope John XXIII who convened the Second Vatican Council. On September 11, 1962, just a month before the opening of the first session of Vatican II, Pope John declared: "In the face of the undeveloped countries, the church is, and wants to be, the church of all, and especially the church of the poor " (Pope John XXIII, 1961, p. xxvi).

The next pope, Paul VI, goes even further in spelling out a strategy for implementing the preferential option for the poor. Even as early as 1971, before the phrase had been coined in Latin America, Pope Paul offers this paraphrase: "In teaching us charity, the Gospel instructs us in the preferential respect due to the poor and the special situation they have in society: the more fortunate should renounce some of their rights so as to place their goods more generously at the service of others" (Pope Paul VI, 1971, par 23).

In such social encyclicals as *Populorum Progressio* (1967) and *Evangelii Nuntiandi* (1975), Paul VI offered social analyses that documented the necessity of profound reforms in social relations. The scope of his suggestions for rigorous corrective measures to benefit the poor knew no bounds, reaching to the international economic system, political procedures, land reform and even the church's own methods of evangelization. The writings he left behind reveal that Pope Paul was a surprisingly prophetic advocate of a progressive agenda marked by a serious commitment to inculturation. He championed a model of development that included a felicitous blend of principles such as enhanced popular participation and liberation of the poor masses of humanity.

Within four months of ascending to the papacy, John Paul II found himself in Mexico, visiting some of the world's poorest neighborhoods (an impressive undertaking he would repeat in Brazil eighteen months later). The first of his many overseas papal travels was primarily for the purpose of presiding over the opening of the Third General Conference of CELAM (*Consejo Episcopal Latinoamericano*), the plenary council of Latin American bishops that met in Puebla, Mexico, from January 27 to February 13, 1979. The words he spoke on several occasions in Mexico—in the homilies at festive masses in Puebla, in an address to the indigenous peoples of nearby provinces, and in a formal Opening Address on January 28 (Eagleson & Sharper, 1979, par. 23) left no doubt that this new pontiff was deeply concerned about the plight of the world's poor, and that he was thoroughly committed to structural changes to benefit the least advantaged. For example, in addressing the people of Oaxaca, John Paul refers to the concern of his predecessor Paul VI:

> With him I would like to reiterate—with an even stronger emphasis in my voice if that were possible—that the present pope wishes to be in solidarity with your cause, which is the cause of the humble people, the poor people. . . . The pope chooses to be your voice, the voice of those who cannot speak or who have been silenced. He wishes to be the conscience of consciences, an invitation to action, to make up for lost time, which has frequently been a time

of prolonged sufferings and unsatisfied hopes (Pope John Paul II, 1979a, p. 82).

To be sure, John Paul II continued to be the voice of orthodoxy (right belief, or doctrine) as well as an advocate of orthopraxis (right conduct of the faith, particularly as regards social justice). On the same trip to Mexico, he issued frequent caveats about the proper understanding of the church's advocacy of social reform, reminding Catholics that, precisely as faithful believers, their mission to social justice must be grounded in authentic Christology, ecclesiology and appropriate theological categories. In so doing, the pope echoed the reservations of many observers regarding the possibility that the church might be growing entirely too political through its endorsement of social movements and its calls for sweeping change. Thus, in the very same Opening Address at Puebla in which John Paul repeatedly invoked the concept of "liberation" and praised local church efforts to "care for the poor, the sick, the dispossessed, the neglected and the oppressed" (July 13, 2004, 1979b, p. 69), he also warned against the potential reduction of transcendent values associated with the Kingdom of God to immanent programs for social reform:

> Emptied of its full content, the Kingdom of God is understood in a rather secularist sense: i.e., we do not arrive at the Kingdom through faith and membership in the Church but rather merely by structural change and sociopolitical involvement. Where there is a certain kind of commitment and praxis for justice, there the Kingdom is already present. This view forgets that "the Church receives the mission to proclaim and to establish among all peoples the kingdom of Christ and of God. She becomes on earth the initial building forth of that kingdom" (Pope John Paul II, 1979b, p. 62).

This cautious balancing of support for the preferential option for the poor, on one hand, and insistence on a framework of orthodox church teachings, on the other hand, would continue to characterize the social teachings of the entire papacy of John Paul II. His social encyclicals, particularly *Sollicitudo Rei Socialis* in 1987 and *Centesimus Annus* in 1991, are punctuated by frequent references to this principle, although John Paul seems to prefer alternative phrasings such as "preferential yet not exclusive love for the poor" and "option or love of preference for the poor" (Pope John Paul II, 1987, par. 42). John Paul clearly accepts the concept as a summary and symbol of the tradition of Catholic social teaching and as an important motivating principle for social involvement. He repeatedly links it to the virtue of solidarity, a favorite leitmotiv of his social thought. At the same time, John Paul takes pain to distinguish the option for the poor from any type of Marxist class struggle. In keeping with traditional Catholic social theory, which emphasizes harmony and organic relations among all sectors of human society rather than a world view where conflict predominates, John Paul rejects any approach that excludes a social group, rich or poor, from the ministry and concern of the church. The church must continue to serve the world always as an agent of reconciliation, so it must not in any crass way take sides.

This attempt to maintain a carefully balanced approach in potentially highly polarized situations helps explain the writing of two important documents in the mid-1980s that treated controversial issues regarding liberation theology. In 1984, the Vatican Congregation for the Doctrine of the Faith (under the leadership of Cardinal Joseph Ratzinger but clearly with the close oversight of the pope himself) issued its *Instruction on Certain Aspects of the Theology of Liberation* (Vatican Congregation for the Doctrine of the Faith, 1984). Two years later, the same Congregation published its *Instruction on Christian Freedom and Liberation* (Vatican Congregation for the Doctrine of the Faith, 1986). By way of summary, suffice it to say that the two documents offer a carefully nuanced endorsement of liberation theology, provided that its central themes are rightly understood and articulated. The first document focuses on correcting potential misinterpretations of the message of such themes as option for the poor, while the second provides a more positive (although still highly qualified) assessment of the contributions of liberation theology to the life of the church. The writing of these instructions further illustrates how the church magisterium during the papacy of John Paul II avoided adopting wholesale either the approach of the progressives or of the conservatives. It sought to bridge the gap amidst some fiercely contested landscape, of which the option for the poor was a key feature.

A Preferential Option for the Poor

A helpful way of viewing the work of the conference of Latin American bishops (in all of its meetings since Vatican II, but especially in the 1968 meeting in Medellin, Colombia, and the 1979 meeting in Puebla, Mexico) is to recognize that the bishops from these troubled lands have been attempting to apply to their local contexts the call of Vatican II to take on the church's constant "duty of scrutinizing the signs of the times and interpreting them in the light of the gospel" (Pope Paul VI, 1992, par. 4). To apply the option for the poor to Latin America necessitates coming to grips with a sharply divided social context, where a great gulf separates a rich ruling elite from the poor masses who are unjustly denied opportunities for upward mobility. The bishops of the United States face a completely different set of challenges in their task of evangelization for justice. A nation like the United States, where the dominant ethos is that of a large and prosperous middle class, and where social mobility is more generally attainable, requires a different approach to the task of portraying and addressing the task of social justice. Remarkably, the concept of preferential option for the poor has nevertheless emerged as entirely relevant in this, the most affluent society in the history of the world. In their longest and most prominent treatment of social justice, the 1986 pastoral letter *Economic Justice for All*, the US bishops speak frequently of the option for the poor. The phrase itself is mentioned nine times in this document, and the general notion of solidarity with the least advantaged members of society pervades the entire 365-paragraph letter.

In this document the bishops make the point that America's prosperity does not excuse us from the moral obligation to make special provisions for the poor. Those with the greatest need require the greatest response, and the automatic workings of our market economy do not guarantee adequate opportunities for social advancement. Trickle-down approaches to economics are not enough; the dire poverty that persists in our "land of plenty" is unacceptable and must be addressed through deliberate commitments to structural change in our institutions, beyond whatever voluntary charitable efforts Americans might make. In their resulting emphasis on extending opportunities to the underprivileged, the bishops echo a sentiment expressed by the Nobel laureate economist, Amartya Sen: "Equal consideration for all may demand very unequal treatment in favor of the disadvantaged" (Sen, 1991, p. 1).

Very early in the letter, the bishops propose three questions that constitute a yardstick for measuring the justice of any economy: "What does the economy do *for* people? What does it do *to* people? And how do people *participate* in it?" (United States Catholic Bishops, 1992, ch. 1, par. 1). A particularly important section of chapter two of the bishops' letter is entitled "Moral Priorities for the Nation" and includes these insights:

> The obligation to provide justice for all means that the poor have the single most urgent economic claim on the conscience of the nation. ... As individuals and as a nation, therefore, we are called to make a fundamental "option for the poor". ... The prime purpose of this special commitment to the poor is to enable them to become active participants in the life of society. It is to enable all persons to share in and contribute to the common good. The "option for the poor," therefore, is not an adversarial slogan that pits one class or group against another (United States Catholic Bishops, 1992, pars. 86-88).

While a context of relative overall prosperity might call for a more subtle understanding of the content of the option for the poor, the US bishops' letter demonstrates what we saw at the outset: that the option for the poor involves an epistemological step (seeing reality through the eyes of the poor) even before it leads us to consider the concrete social engagements that result from commitment to such an option.

IV. A Case Study in Institutionalizing an Option for the Poor: The Jesuits of Latin America

In the remaining space, let us examine the experience of one group of men who succeeded in placing the poor at the center of their vision and who undertook institutional changes to put themselves on the side of the poor in practical (and eventually extremely costly) ways. The Jesuits of Latin America are heirs to nearly five hundred years of

A Preferential Option for the Poor

Jesuit history and spirituality, extending back to the life journey of their founder, St. Ignatius of Loyola (1491-1556). Ignatius may be said to have undergone a conversion that led to a distinctive type of option for the poor. Much like St. Francis of Assisi, Gautama Buddha and many other religious virtuosi, he gave up a life of privilege and honor (the Loyolas were an affluent Basque family of minor nobility, and Ignatius himself had been a courtier at a royal palace) in order to offer humble service to the church.

At a very early moment in the life of the Society of Jesus, the religious order that Ignatius founded, evidence of a distinctive Jesuit style of option for the poor became evident. In the winter of 1539-40, while Ignatius and his ten early companions were in Rome waiting for definitive approval and mission of their religious institute by Pope Paul III, they found themselves engaged in a most intriguing series of apostolic labors for social improvement. Ignatius' expressed desire to work directly with the poor for the betterment of the social outcasts of Rome encountered resistance and frustration at every turn until a gradual realization dawned on him. The conversion of the powerful elites (through preaching, teaching and hearing confessions) to a sense of greater social responsibility emerged as an even more efficacious instrument of social change than the small band's customary direct ministries to the sick, imprisoned and destitute. While still maintaining proximity to the poor (the earliest Jesuits themselves were constantly on the brink of utter indigence), the mission to the powerful became a key instrument of social improvement and institutional change. Ignatius' efforts to reintegrate prostitutes into respectable society, his struggle to foster greater legal rights for the long-oppressed Jews of Rome, his desire to establish more reliable systems of credit and alms distribution to the disabled—all proved to depend upon simultaneous work with both rich and poor. A contemporary French historian familiar with the writings of Ignatius and his companions describes this dynamic thus:

> In all these documents, one can sense an attention, discreet but clear, to the institutional dimensions of problems. Ignatius encouraged the foundation of cooperative lending institutions. The "works of piety" of the Jesuits in favor of the poor tended to take on something of the nature of a partial reform of society. They may seem timid

to us. That age, however, had not yet conceived the idea of action on social structures as such, nor did it have the mental categories to think in those terms. But their "way of proceeding" moved in that direction, notably in a reorganization of medieval confraternities, orienting them toward social action which was not uniquely "charitable" (Demoustier, 1990, p. 16).

It was the same drive to deal not just with the effects but the causes of poverty that led the Jesuits in 1548 to do something they had earlier agreed not to undertake—to establish (in Messina, Sicily) a college for lay students. This marked the Jesuits' first involvement in a school that went beyond the formation needs of their own members. The entire subsequent history of Jesuit education springs from the incipient institutional analysis that led Ignatius to pursue the "multiplier effect" for his efforts. Ignatius discerned opportunities to reap greater benefits precisely for the poorest of society by focusing some apostolic energies toward the more elite classes whose lives could be touched, in the case of educational institutions, by the Jesuit schoolmasters. At Jesuit schools, the potential social benefits were many: social barriers were broken when the rich and poor would mingle; the teachers could model to the affluent students the importance of commitment to the side of the lowly; and the tuition-free environment allowed a unique opportunity for upward mobility for the lower classes.

After centuries of less explicit attention to the mission to social justice, the Jesuits' self-understanding underwent a dramatic renewal in the 1960's. Another fiery Basque, this one named Pedro Arrupe, was elected in 1965 to lead the Jesuit order. In 1966 Arrupe addressed the superiors of the Latin American provinces of the Society of Jesus, reminding them of the contradiction between the socioeconomic inequality of their homelands and the gospel message, challenging them thus: "From this situation rises the moral obligation of the Society of Jesus to rethink all its ministries and every form of its apostolates to see if they really offer a response to the urgent priorities that justice and social equality call for" (Arrupe, 1966, p. 791). A subsequent meeting of Arrupe with the same group in Rio de Janeiro (May 6-14, 1968) produced a final statement in which the provincials committed to transforming their institutions into instruments for social change. "We promise to work for bold reforms that will radically transform existing structures to promote social peace" (Arrupe, 1966, pp. 49-50).

Business as usual would not be good enough, at least not for the Latin American Jesuits. As the post-Vatican II church as a whole was for the first time considering the preferential option for the poor, Jesuit schools and other institutions were being challenged to renew their commitment to the poor.

V. Paying the Price

At this juncture, the story could be told in a number of ways. The broadest telling would mention the influence of the subsequent General Congregations, the worldwide legislative assemblies of the Jesuit order. In 1974-5, General Congregation 32 issued a famous decree declaring: "The mission of the Society of Jesus today is the service of faith, of which the promotion of justice is an absolute requirement" *(Decrees of the 31st and 32nd General Congregations of the Society of Jesus,* 1977, p. 411). Subsequent General Congregations (number 33 in 1983 and number 34 in 1995) reaffirmed this direction, as did Arrupe's successor Peter-Hans Kolvenbach in his numerous addresses on justice and education and their interrelation. [2] But the case study that demonstrates the preferential option for the poor most dramatically involves just a few Jesuits in one of the world's smallest nations and least influential regions: El Salvador in Central America.

The Universidad Centroamericana José Simeón Cañas (UCA for short) was established in San Salvador, the capital of El Salvador, on September 15, 1965. From the beginning, its mission was more than just the usual, somewhat bland goal of a generic university, namely to promote the search for truth and knowledge. Its Jesuit founders included in its original charter the task of bringing Christian inspiration and energy to the very divided Salvadoran society. Even to state from the start that its aspirations included goals like development, social transformation and real enjoyment of fundamental human rights was provocative, for El Salvador was (and continues to be even after decades of civil war and low-intensity conflict) very much an oligarchic society, where the rights of only a small elite class count for much. The UCA positioned itself to play a leading role as a force of cultural resistance within the tumultuous recent history of El Salvador.

Charles Beirne has amply documented the gradual gestation of increasingly bold social analysis and outreach on the part of the UCA in the early decades of its existence (Beirne, 1996).[3] Only the briefest of summaries of the factors that make the UCA such a distinctive and prophetic institution can be recounted here. Certainly, one key factor was bold leadership, including the rectorships (the equivalent of presidencies in American colleges) of Luis Achaerandio from 1969-75 and later Ignacio Ellacuría in the 1980s. Faculty included extremely dedicated and mission-driven lay people and Jesuits, including outstandingly brilliant members of the order (Jon Sobrino, Ignacio Martín-Baró and Ignacio Ellacuría, among others) who had been designated by their superiors for special studies in the United States and Europe for the express purpose of filling high profile jobs at the UCA. This investment in talent and human resources was a prerequisite for successful involvement in this educational work.

A second factor that facilitated the enactment of a preferential option for the poor on the part of the UCA was a clear and direct set of institutional policies. The charter, bylaws and composition of the board of directors of the UCA all fostered hiring, promotion and admission policies that sent a clear message that the university's goals went far beyond narrowly conceived professionalism and academic achievement. The university emphasized social vision and a commitment to transformation of social structures, not satisfied to reward mere competence on the part of its students and faculty. Research projects that focused on issues of justice, poverty and human rights were favored over merely technical ones that did nothing to challenge the oppressive status quo of the nation. Even the architecture and layout of the campus was deliberately selected to encourage a mingling of personnel and a cross-fertilization of departments intended to overcome the tendency of faculty to isolate themselves into quarreling academic fiefdoms. But it was a distinctive egalitarian financial policy that most clearly set the UCA apart from other universities in poor countries.

> Anxious for financial security but determined to admit students who could not afford to pay even low tuition, the UCA adopted a differentiated tuition structure (*cuotas diferenciadas*) in which students pay according to their means, and a unique salary scale that

closes the income gaps among personnel of various ranks (Beirne, 1996, p. 91).

Besides these internal dynamics of the functioning of the UCA, the university was able to publicize its social commitments to a large external audience through its numerous publications (e.g., *Estudios Centroamericanos*, a scholarly journal run by the UCA), a third significant factor that multiplied the awareness and effects of UCA's option for the poor. Everybody in San Salvador knew what the Jesuits and the UCA stood for in its teaching, research and social outreach. Editorials in UCA publications as well as research projects that proved embarrassing to sitting governments led periodically to serious tensions and even several instances when the military, in a foreboding show of force calculated to intimidate intellectual critics of the privileges of the elite class, occupied the Jesuit campus during the 1970s and 1980s.

A fourth and final factor in the UCA's dedication to its mission emerges as an immediate corollary of the above. It concerns how the UCA related to those who became its critics, both internally and externally. Some internal dissent from faculty and administrators was inevitable, but more often it took the form of indifference rather than outright opposition. Those who did not adopt an option for the poor and did not seek to enact it through the life of the university generally found other venues for their professional work or study. More significant was external opposition, particularly from the oligarchy that controlled the government, most other social institutions and often even church structures in El Salvador. Voices denouncing the work of the UCA were heard especially loud whenever university research or advocacy touched sensitive current issues such as the conduct of the war against the guerrillas, foreign policy, fraudulent elections, nationwide strikes, land reform, population policy and similar contested issues in the Salvadoran context. The best way to summarize the UCA's strategy for preserving its preferential option despite opposition is simply to affirm three truths: 1) the UCA never hesitated to take sides on social issues; (2) it allowed its positions to be guided by what in the long term would be best for the poor majority of the Salvadoran people; and (3) it was willing to pay the price for boldly staking out its positions.

These three points require some clarification. The Spanish word *universitariamente* is a felicitous adverb that contextualizes the first two points with great acuity. Ignacio Ellacuría and Jon Sobrino, among the most prominent of the UCA Jesuits, used this word frequently to modify how their school proceeded. In all its undertakings, UCA sought to engage in social action "in a university fashion." Engagement in politics and support for social reform movements were not off-limits, as long as UCA's self-understanding remained larger than any given action or particular partisan involvement. The ultimate goal was structural transformation of society toward greater justice, and any number of means might be judged acceptable for a university community whose "horizon of concern" remains the poor majority, in this case the national reality of the Salvadoran people.[4] The UCA Jesuits not only acted on this set of institutional priorities, but they also made frequent attempts to explain their actions to a variety of audiences who might learn from their experience. [5]

The third point above, about the willingness of the UCA community to "pay the price" of its provocative stances and actions, might be interpreted as referring to mundane items such as the opportunity cost of donations not secured from conservative rich benefactors. But the most serious ramifications of "paying the price" have already been eloquently expressed in the lives and deaths of many members of the UCA community, most dramatically the six Jesuits assassinated at their residence on UCA campus on November 16, 1989. These men and two female employees died at the hands of the Atlacatl Battalion of the El Salvadoran army. Beirne captures poignantly the linkage between the work and the deaths of the UCA martyrs:

> The university refused merely to prepare students professionally without a social vision, because that would perpetuate the oppressive structures that held the majority in subjugation and injustice.
> ... The proponents of this university model were not naive; they realized the consequences of their commitment and they were willing to pay the price, both on a day-to-day basis and in the ultimate sacrifice of their lives. . . . They recognized the national reality as they found it: a country with a privileged minority enjoying affluence at the expense of the vast majority . . . and it took a stand at the side of the majority (Beirne, 1996, pp. 228-29).

VI. The Task Ahead: Applying the Lessons of this Case Study to US Health Care and Health Sciences Systems

Examining this case study offers a glimpse at what the preferential option for the poor looks like in a specific institutional context. However, it obviously remains a situation very different from the distinctive challenges facing health care provision in the US Before useful lessons are appropriated, a certain amount of "translation of idioms" must be undertaken in the interest of crossing the divide into our own culture and field of inquiry. Many questions quickly arise: is it likely that any version of the preferential option for the poor will ever exert broad appeal in a culture as individualistic and achievement-oriented in its ethos as is ours? How precisely can we expect large and pluralistic institutions such as American health care providers to act with the requisite unity of purpose? Are established measures (such as the Catholic Hospital Association's 1991 decision to develop "social accountability budgets" to assess actual service to America's poor) to benefit the least advantaged in US society best viewed as harbingers of change or relics from a romanticized past of richer social concern? Will we ever be able to say about our health care and health sciences institutions what the martyr Ellacuría said about the UCA: "The university of Christian inspiration is not a place of security, selfish interests, honor or profit, and worldly splendor, but a place of sacrifice, personal commitment and renunciation" (Ellacuría, 1991)?

The task of answering these questions constitutes an ambitious research agenda for health care ethicists, policy analysts and education specialists. It is an agenda with great potential rewards as well as considerable costs, both predictable and unanticipated in nature. The pattern by which we can learn from the case study of the UCA Jesuits is clearly articulated by Ellacuría when he spells out the threefold challenge presented by liberation theology's adoption of the preferential option for the poor. The first challenge is to gain *insight* into the present situation (the "noetic" task, in his terminology). The second "moment" is to spark and sustain a *commitment* (the "ethical" task). The third stage is to take action (the task of "praxis") in the struggle for justice.[6] These steps, sometimes summarized as the engagement of "the head, heart and hands," emerge as an invariant pattern of how to make progress toward institutionalizing a preferential option for the poor.

The central figures in our case study of the UCA demonstrated what this transformation looks like for a university in a Central American context. They pioneered the search for how to conduct a preferential option for the poor "in a university way." It is now up to others, using this groundwork, to explore the features of a transformation toward an option for the poor in the challenging context of the health care and health sciences systems in the US and elsewhere and carry out this task "in a health-care-system way."

Notes

[1] Theologian Donal Dorr, for example, entitled his survey of Catholic social teaching since 1891, *Option for the poor: A hundred years of Vatican social thought*. (1992). Maryknoll, NY: Orbis Books.

[2] See for example "The Jesuit University in the Light of the Ignatian Charism," address to the International Meeting of Jesuit Higher Education, Rome, 27 May 2001; also "The Service of Faith and the Promotion of Justice in American Jesuit Higher Education," address at Santa Clara University, 6 October 2000, reprinted in *Studies in the Spirituality of Jesuits*, vol. 35, no. 1 (January 2001): 13-29.

[3] See Beirne, (1996). Beirne's knowledge of the history of the UCA comes first-hand, as he was one of the Jesuits who filled vacant posts there after the November 16, 1989, assassinations.

[4] This phrasing permeates Ignacio Ellacuría's impressive essay "Is a Different Kind of University Possible?," first published in Spanish in 1975 in *Estudios Centroamericanos*. A translation (by Phillip Berryman) appears as chapter 9 in J Hassett and H Lacey (eds.). (1991). *Towards a society that serves its people: The intellectual contribution of El Salvador's murdered Jesuits*. Washington, DC: Georgetown University Press.

[5] See, for example, a talk delivered by Ellacuría on 12 June 1982 at the graduation exercises of Santa Clara University in California, entitled "The Task of a Christian University." It appears in J Sobrino et al (1990). *Companions of Jesus: The Jesuit martyrs of El Salvador*. NY: Orbis Books.

[6] For a detailed treatment of this theological method, see Ignacio Ellacuría, "Utopia and Prophecy in Latin America," in J Sobrino and I Ellacuría (eds.). *Mysterium liberationis: fundamental concepts of liberation theology*.

References

Arrupe, P, SJ, (1966). On the social apostolate in Latin America. *Acta Romana*, 14(6) 791.

———. et al. (1996). Communiqué of the Latin American provincials, March 1966. In Beirne, SJ, C, *Jesuit education and social change in El Salvador*. NY: Garland Publishing, Inc.

Beirne, SJ, C, (1996). *Jesuit education and social change in El Salvador*. NY: Garland Publishing, Inc.

Decrees of the 31st and 32nd General Congregations of the Society of Jesus (1977). St. Louis: Institute of Jesuit Sources.

Demoustier, A, SJ (1990). The first companions and the poor, *Studies in the Spirituality of Jesuits*, 21(2).

Dorr, D (1992). *Option for the poor: A hundred years of Vatican social thought*. Maryknoll, NY: Orbis Books.

Ellacuría, I (1991). Is a different kind of university possible? In J Hassett & H Lacey (eds.). *Toward a society that serves its people: The intellectual contribution of El Salvador's murdered Jesuits*. Washington, DC: Georgetown University Press.

———. (1993). Utopia and prophecy in Latin America. In J Sobrino SJ & I Ellacuría, SJ, (eds.). (1993). *Mysterium liberationis: Fundamental concepts of liberation theology*. Maryknoll, NY: Orbis Books.

———, & J Sobrino, SJ and I Ellacuría, SJ (eds.). (1993). *Mysterium liberationis: Fundamental concepts of liberation theology*. Maryknoll, NY: Orbis Books.

J Eagleson & P Scharper (eds.). (1979). *Puebla and beyond: Documentation and commentary*. Maryknoll, NY: Orbis Books.

Gutierrez, G (1993). Option for the poor. In I Ellacuira, SJ & J Sobrino, SJ (eds.). (1993). *Mysterium liberationis: Fundamental concepts of liberation theology*. Maryknoll, NY: Orbis Books.

Kolvenbach, SJ, PH, (2001). The Jesuit university in the light of the Ignatian charism. Address to the International Meeting of Jesuit Higher Education, Rome, 27 May.

———. (2001). The service of faith and the promotion of justice in American Jesuit higher education. Address at Santa Clara University, 6 October 2000. In *Studies in the Spirituality of Jesuits*, 35(1) 13-29.

Pope John XXIII (1962). Allocution of September 11. In Gutiérrez, G (1988). Introduction to the revised edition. *A theology of liberation, fifteenth anniversary edition*. Maryknoll, NY: Orbis Books.

Pope John Paul II (1979a) Address to the Indians of Oaxaca and Chiapas. In J Eagleson & P Scharper (eds.). *Puebla and beyond: documentation and commentary*. Maryknoll, NY: Orbis Books.

———. (1979b). Opening address at the Puebla conference, 28 January 1979. In J Eagleson & P Scharper (eds.). *Puebla and beyond: Documentation and commentary*. Maryknoll, NY: Orbis Books. 0

———. (1987). *Sollicitudo rei socialis*. In DJ O'Brien & A Shannon (eds.). *Catholic social thought: The documentary heritage*. Maryknoll, NY: Orbis Books.

Pope Paul VI (1992). *Gaudium et spes*. In DJ O'Brien and A Shannon (eds.). *Catholic social thought: The documentary heritage*. Maryknoll, NY: Orbis Books.

———. (1975). *Evangelii nuntiandi*. In DJ O'Brien & A Shannon (eds.). *Catholic social thought: The documentary heritage*. Maryknoll, NY: Orbis Books.

———. (1971). *Octogesima adveniens*. Apostolic Letter of May 14.

———. (1967). *Populorum progressio*. In DJ O'Brien & A Shannon (eds.). *Catholic social thought: The documentary heritage*. Maryknoll, NY: Orbis Books.

———. (1964). *Lumen Gentium*. (1990). In: NP Tanner (ed.). *Decrees of the ecumenical councils*. 2 vol. London: Sheed & Ward: Washington: Georgetown University Press.

Puebla Final Document (1979). *Puebla and beyond: Documentation and commentary*. Latin American Bishops meeting in Puebla, Mexico. In J Eagleson & P Scharper (eds.). (1979). Maryknoll, NY: Orbis Books.

Sen, A (1991). *Inequality reexamined*. Cambridge, MA: Harvard University Press.

United Nations Development Program (1999). *1999 United Nations Development Report*. NY: Oxford University Press.

United States Catholic Bishops (1992). *Economic justice for all*. In DJ O'Brien & A Shannon (eds.). *Catholic social thought: The documentary heritage*. Maryknoll, NY: Orbis Books.

Vatican Congregation for the Doctrine of the Faith (1984). Instruction on certain aspects of the theology of liberation. *Origins*, 14(13) 193, 195-204.

———. (1986). Instruction on Christian freedom and liberation. *Origins*, 15 (44) 713, 715-28.

World Synod of Catholic Bishops (1971). Justice in the world. In DJ O'Brien & A Shannon (eds.). *Catholic social thought: The documentary heritage*. Maryknoll, NY: Orbis Books.

Part II

Justice as the Hallmark of Jesuit Health Sciences Education

5. Walter Burghardt, SJ

Biblical Justice and "The Cry of the Poor": Jesuit Medicine and the Third Millennium

EDITORIAL NOTE: The following is the literal text of a lecture presented by Father Burghardt at Georgetown University Medical Center on March 17, 1994. His was the last in a series of four lectures entitled "The Jesuit Tradition and Medicine." All four lectures were first published in Huey (1994). Father Burghardt's lecture is reprinted here with the permission of both the author and Georgetown University Medical Center.

This current series of lectures within the Medical Center has a general title: "The Jesuit Tradition and Medicine." The Jesuit tradition. In harmony with that expression, three distinguished Jesuits have traced for you the exciting story of Jesuit medicine in three engaging directions. In November 1992, John Padberg summarized brilliantly the Jesuit involvement in medicine through 452 years: who and what and why and how. In April 1993, Georgetown's own class-act historian R. Emmett Curran, detailed the first hundred years in the fascinating history of medicine at Georgetown, "From 'Sundown College' to Medical Center." In October 1993, Edwin Cassem recalled in delightfully personal accents our more recent tradition in psychiatry.

Indispensable stories, with inspiring addenda on the human, Christian, Catholic significance of it all. But tradition in its genuine understanding is not some musty museum piece, "This is the way we've always done it." That benighted bit of balderdash proves only one thing: This is the way we've always done it. Tradition in its richness is a living, throbbing, thrilling reality: the best of the past, infused with the insights of the present, with a view to a richer, more catholic (small c) future. The best of a past; for (no news to you) not everything "Jesuitical" that happened in four and half centuries deserves to endure. The insights of the present; for one encouraging aspect of the human, including the Jesuit, is our capacity to grow, to develop, to improve. A richer future; for the creative and imaginative scenario you set up will influence profoundly, perhaps determine definitively, the shape of our nation's health in the third millennium.

What do I propose to do? In the light of the tradition, I want to read the "signs of the times," our times, and in the light of that reading, I want to suggest what I should like to see, not in technological advance but in the men and women whose privilege and burden it will be to touch technology to the human person, to help men, women and children to live holy lives more wholly in the image and likeness of God—perhaps in the image and likeness of the Jesus whose mission and gift it was to heal wholly.

I. Signs of the Times

First then, the signs of the times. What do I mean? By "signs of the times" I mean "the main characteristics and events, including secular ones, of each age and place, which reveal the actions and will of God in history and in peoples" (McGrath, 1986, p. 325). Not the Lord God thundering to us as of old from Mount Sinai; not Jesus addressing us once again from a hillside or a boat. Rather, God speaking to us through the events of history, in the lives of living people. Not all the signs; simply those I see as addressing, challenging the men and women whose day-to-day living is the health of others. For you and your ministry of health, I shall suggest three signs of the times: (1) the close connection between illness and social ills; (2) the cries of the socially ill, the so-called "poor"; and (3) the resurgence of rugged individualism.

A. Connection between Social Ills and Illness

A significant sign of our times is an ever-increasing awareness of the close connection between illness and social ills. New York's Governor Mario Cuomo put it pungently: "Illness does not occur in a vacuum... the roots of illness are usually deeply implanted in homelessness, in poverty, in other persistent social ills" (Cuomo, 1991, p. 126). He went on to write:

> Health, perhaps more than any other aspect of our lives, depends upon the interconnectedness of everything else we are and do. The very word "health" has the same root as "whole." It denotes an integrity based upon the immensely complex synergy that includes the workings of the human body and all the external forces that affect it. Health is not given, nor taken away, in a vacuum.... the relationship between illness, sickness, and physical frailty on the one hand, and poverty on the other, is not just a grotesque coincidence. It is causal. It is real. It is historic (Cuomo, 1991, pp. 127-8).

It was in this context that Kevin Cahill, senior member of the New York City Board of Health, could remind us:

> The "public" served by the public health system is increasingly the disenfranchised, the uninsured, the impoverished, the homeless, the aged, the addicted. Failing their needs is more than morally indefensible in our "new world order"; it threatens the health of all. For as surely as an untreated tuberculous lesion will cavitate the lungs of a homeless vagrant, so too will the deadly mist of his infection disseminate through every social and economic class, among innocent fellow riders in the subway, or passengers in the elevator and, inevitably, from child to child in the classrooms of our city (Cahill, 1991, p. 126).

B. Cries to the Poor

Given the interconnectedness between illness and the socially ill, a second, related sign of the times stems from the "cries of the poor." By "the poor" I mean not simply the economically disadvantaged.

You might recall who "the poor" are in Scripture, in God's own Book. The poverty-stricken, of course; but others as well. Poor was the leper, ostracized from society, excluded from normal association with others, compelled often to live outside his town. Poor was the widow, who could not inherit from her husband, was an obvious victim for creditors, had no defender at law. Poor were the orphans with no parents to love them. Poor was the woman caught in adultery, to be stoned according to the law of Moses. Poor were those of a lower class oppressed by the powerful. Poor, in brief, were the socially ill.

Who are the poor that cry out to us in our time? Here are four examples. First, the cries of our children. One of every five little ones grows up hungry in the richest nation on earth, a poverty rate more than double that of any other major industrialized nation; 40,000 each year do not survive to celebrate their first birthday. Every 26 seconds a child runs away from home, every 47 seconds a child is abused or neglected, every 67 seconds a teenager has a baby, every seven minutes a boy or girl is arrested for drug abuse, every 36 minutes a child is killed or injured by a gun. The head of Covenant House dedicated her 1991 book, *God's Lost Children*, "to the 1,000,000 homeless children who slept on America's streets last year, scared, cold, hungry, alone, and most of all, desperate to find someone who cares."[1] At least 30,000 children in the US have lost one or both parents to AIDS; that number will triple in the next seven years.[2]

In our own District of Columbia, a dismaying trend has come to light. Children in Washington are planning their own funerals: how they want to look, how be dressed, where be waked. They simply do not believe they will be around very long, have every reason to suspect they will not grow up. Where they play, coke and crack are homicidal kings. In the past five years, 224 of their childhood friends have died from gunfire. Some were deliberate targets, others just happened to be there, at least one lay in a cradle. And so the living little ones have begun planning for the worst, as if their own murders are inevitable, as if their own dreams will surely be just as cruelly cut short.[3]

And across the world, do you know how many children will die this decade alone, the '90's; most from diseases we know how to prevent? One hundred and fifty million!

Biblical Justice and the Cry of the Poor

Second, the cries of the elderly. What does our dominant American culture glorify? Youth, strength, beauty. The ideal of aging? Not to seem to age at all. Bob Hope and Eva Gabor, Ronald Reagan and Mother Teresa, Cary Grant and Grandma Moses, George Burns and Jacqueline Kennedy, Paul Newman and Katherine Hepburn—here is eternal youth. If after 60 or 65 you can continue a productive career, stroke a tennis ball, straddle a Honda, satisfy a sexual partner, then your aging is ideal.

Most Americans, however, do not age so gracefully, so creatively, so productively. Most sexagenarians, practically all septuagenarians, are "retired." In our culture, to be retired is to be literally "useless." The aged rarely serve a practical purpose; they don't "do" anything. Not only are they irrelevant to big business, big government, big labor, big military, big education; they are a drain on the economy. Whether glowing with health or in a permanent vegetative state, they use up medical resources, medical miracles, that could benefit the useful members of society. The "new boys [and girls] on the block," economic man an economic woman, draw their knowledge and wisdom from computers, not from the hoary stories of the aging. Honor them, naturally—till they become an economic liability meriting a merciful injection. Respect for elders, of course; but life in the same house with grandpa and grandma? It simply would not work. Too wide a gap between the generations; the old folk are not "with it." On the whole, a nursing home makes better American sense. And there they sit, watching and waiting: watching TV's "Married—with Children" and waiting for someone they carried in their womb to visit and "watch one hour" (Matthew 26:40) with them.

Third, the cry of our black sisters and brothers. Their cry echoes the cry of Yahweh to Pharaoh, "Let my people go" (Exodus 5:1). Rather than listen to barren statistics, listen to black Sister Thea Bowman, stricken with breast cancer and bone cancer, racing her wheelchair across the country to spread her gospel of universal love, speaking her mind passionately to the bishops of the Catholic church in 1989:

> . . . despite the civil rights movement of the '60s and the socio-educational gains of the '70s, blacks in the '80s are still struggling, still scratching and clawing as the old folks said, still trying to find home in the homeland and home in the church, still struggling to

gain access to equal opportunity.... A disproportionate number of black people are poor. Poverty, deprivation, stunted physical, intellectual and spiritual growth—I don't need to tell you this, but I want to remind you, more than a third of the black people that live in the United States live in poverty, the kind of poverty that lacks basic necessity.... I'm talking about old people who have worked hard all their lives and don't have money for adequate food or shelter or medical care.... I'm talking about children who can never have equal access and equal opportunity because poverty doomed them to low birth weight and retardation and unequal opportunity for education.... Black children are twice as likely as white children to be born prematurely, to suffer from low birth weight, to live in substandard housing, to have no parent employed. ... One of every 21 black males is murdered. A disproportionate number of our men are dying of suicide and AIDS and drug abuse and low self-esteem (Cepress, 1989, p. 31).

Fourth, the cry of the AIDS-afflicted. For many Americans, AIDS (Acquired Immune Deficiency Syndrome) is God's own plague on the promiscuous. It is indeed a fact that more Americans die of AIDS each year than died in the entire Vietnam War. It is a fact that the most technologically advanced society in history faces a plague in the late-twentieth century that mocks our medical ingenuity. But the AIDS-afflicted raise cries that must not only challenge our minds but rend our hearts. I heard those cries with exquisite agony from an Anglican minister addressing the 73rd Assembly of the Catholic Health Association of the United States: "I stand here with you—as a brother to you, a churchman, a man with AIDS. A man who regrets nothing of the love and goodness he has known, who stops now to notice flowers, children at play. ...A man who loves his church from his heart, from every molecule in him" (*Catholic Health World*, 1988, p. 1).

He then unfolded a chilling true story of a fox hunt wherein 600 men, women, and children in an Ohio county formed a circle five miles across, frightened all the foxes out of their holes, killed them as they forced them into an ever-diminishing circle. Finally, within a circle a few yards across, the remaining foxes lay down, "for they knew not what else to do, But the men and the women knew what to do. They hit these dying wounded with their clubs until they were dead, or they showed their children how to do it." He went on:

> I stand before you today as one weary of running, as one wounded myself, and I say to the churches, the churches first, and then to the government, the silent government, and then to the world: "What have you done to my people? What have you done to your own people—beautiful people . . . ? My people are being destroyed, and your people, and all our people together. Not only by an illness called AIDS, but by a darker illness called hatred. . . . The Christ, Jesus, the compassionate lord of life and lord of more forgiveness and lord of more hope is the one we have vowed to follow and be ultimately guided by. We must tell that to our smugly self-righteous brothers and sisters. . . . For if we do not, their souls will perish in the circle of misunderstanding and scorn they teach so many as they club and scream their disdain for the outsider, the misunderstood, the different. . . . Sadly . . . too many with AIDS have wondered if they had any alternative but to go to the center of the circle and lie down and die. Where are you in that circle? Where are we? Where would Christ be? (*Catholic Health World*, 1988, p. 12).

Cries of the poor indeed. And these do not cry alone. Listen to our women as they cry out against the feminization of poverty, a gender-based division of labor within the family, a powerlessness of women to shape the world in any but a masculine mold, sexual abuse only now beginning to surface in its horrifying extent. Listen to the Hispanic communities, in so many ways second-class citizens, hardly accepted in our Anglo liturgy and life. Listen to our Native Americans, driven from the land they revere, homeless in their own homes, without work, without hope, wracked by alcoholism. Listen to our Jewish sisters and brothers, increasingly fearful as they hear Americans arguing that the Holocaust which consumed six million of their dear ones is a gigantic hoax, never really happened. Listen to the millions of refugees watering the highways of the world with their tears. Listen to the cries from scores of death rows, while most Americans clamor to avenge one killing with another killing, an eye for an eye.

C. Resurgence of Rugged Individualism

Take a third sign of our times. Within recent years respected sociologists have found in our fair land a frightening phenomenon: a resurgence of late nineteenth-century rugged individualism. They find American society moving away from religious man/woman, away from political man/woman, as character ideals. Those ideals were oriented to the public world, the community, the common good, the other. But when the central institution in our society is no longer religion or the political order but the economy, the ideal is now economic man/woman, man and woman in pursuit of private self-interest. Listen to Robert Bellah writing over a decade ago:

> What is significant here is not the Moral Majority... but something that comes closer to being amoral and is in fact a majority. This new middle class believes in the gospel of success 1980 style. It is an ethic of how to get ahead in the corporate, bureaucratic world while maximizing one's private goodies. In the world of the zero-sum society, it is important to get to the well first before it dries up, to look out for number one, to take responsibility for your own life and keep it, while continuing to play the corporate game . . . (Bellah, 1982, p. 652). [4]

This new ideal, we are told, finds its strength in the younger generations. The dominant theme researchers find in young economic man/woman is freedom, autonomy, personal fulfillment. The race is to the swift, the shrewd, the savage; and the devil take the hindmost. Little wonder that in 1986, when Harvard University was celebrating its 350th anniversary, the three top goals declared by the class of 1990 were 1. money, 2. power, 3. reputation.[5] Is Georgetown significantly different?

II. Jesuit Medicine for a Third Millennium

My second main point. What has all this to do with a Jesuit medical tradition, specifically for a third millennium? Not much; just about everything. The central foci here are two sentences I want to recapture from my first point, two insightful observations from Governor Cuomo: (1) "The very word 'health' has the same root as 'whole'"; (2) "The roots of illness are usually deeply implanted in social ills." For these raise and respond to the question why the Society of Jesus has its hands in medicine at all, why it founds medical schools and hospitals. Believe it or not, the reason is not to make money; nor is it to ensure that ailing Jesuits get medical care at a discount. In the remote but still important background lies a divine revelation; in the foreground you have a Jesuit vision. Let me explain.

A. Biblical Justice

The remote revelation may surprise you. It is the biblical idea of justice. You see, when college and university people think of justice, what springs first to their minds is ethical justice: Give to each person what is due to each, what he or she deserves, can claim as a right, because it has written into law or can be proven from philosophy: right to life, decent housing, work, freedom of speech, to be treated with respect, and so on and so forth. Biblical justice recognizes ethical justice, but goes beyond it, above it. Biblical justice is fidelity to relationships, especially those that stem from a covenant with God. God's intent in creating was not to fashion billions of monads, isolated individuals, who might at some point come together through a social contract. God had in view a family, a community, wherein no one could say to any other, "I have no need of you." The Jews were to father the fatherless, mother the motherless, welcome the stranger, not because the orphan an the alien deserved it, but because this was the way God had acted with Israel.

Biblical justice, fidelity to relationships, is summed up in the two great commandments of the law and the gospel—fidelity that goes up and fidelity that goes out: "You shall love the Lord your God with all your heart, and with all your soul, and with all your mind." And "You shall love your neighbor as yourself." This second commandment, Jesus declared, "is like" the first; loving our brothers and sisters is like loving God (Matthew 22:37, 39). And "Love your neighbor as yourself" is not some psychological balance: As much or as little as you love yourself, so much or so little shall you love others. No, the commandment means: Love your sisters and brothers as if they were standing in your shoes.

B. Relationship with a Person

Fidelity to relationships. Here is where the Jesuit tradition in medicine is of supreme significance. For it goes beyond the legal contract between doctor and patient, what Medicare and Blue Cross will pay and the patient is obligated to pay. It passes beyond a doctor's obligation to use all his technical resources, all her medical skill, to excise a tumor, destroy a clot, implant a heart. The Jesuit tradition sees a more profound relationship here. Not primarily with a diseased ovary, with a melanoma. It is a relationship with a person. A person. At its best, a person is a wondrous wedding of mind and heart, of reason and love, of logic and passion, of the divine and the human. But in our dread-full human condition, that wholeness is often shattered by sin, severed by schizophrenia, rent by all manner of hates and hurts, fears and tears, men and women afraid of dying, at times afraid of living. In either case, ideal or dread-full, a person is not an abstraction. In either case, the real, pulsating life I live is never flesh or spirit. It is always and inescapably a man or a woman who is born and dies, loves or hates, gives life or takes it, laughs or cries, dances in sheer delight or winces in unbearable pain.

In fact, the so-called "patient" is always a person-in-process-of-redemption, working out his or her salvation, hoping and perhaps praying that this medical center, this medicine man or woman, might stitch together some of the brokenness in the human composite. A disease is not something objective, outside of me. It is I, as really and existentially part of me as is my hand or my hearing, my faith and my fears, my loves and my deepest yearnings. In illness I work out my destiny as a person: I grow or I diminish, I am spent selflessly for others or selfishly for myself. If disease diminishes me, it diminishes my Christianess; if sickness strengthens me, I take a giant step, or many small steps, toward my salvation.

This tradition, this realization, lays on you frightening demands. As individuals and as a community. As individuals, it means that no one enters your clinic as an object, your medical center as a wrist tag, your operating room as a piece of flesh on a gurney. It is always and everywhere a relationship between two persons, a relationship as intimate as that between a priest and a penitent. And so it calls for a singular wedding of competence and compassion, of knowledge and love. I am not about to turn you into weeping willows, men and women whose hands shake with compassion as you wield the scalpel. I do mean that you share, in some genuine fashion, the lot of the men, women, and children you serve. I mean, you hurt with those who hurt, you weep with those who weep. Whenever a sister or brother dies, you yourself feel diminished. A pertinent, or impertinent, question: Can you say with an ancestor of yours named Hippocrates that you would rather know what sort of person has a disease than what sort of disease a person has?

In different language I am simply commending to you two strong statements from Dr. Bernie Siegel. Profoundly Jewish, past president of the American Holistic Medical Association, a man who labored to make patients aware of their own healing potential, he has authored a remarkable book entitled Love, Medicine, and Miracles. The two statements? (1). "Remember I said love heals. I do not claim love cures everything but it can heal and in the process of healing cures occur also" (Siegel, 1988, p. 57). (2). "I am convinced that unconditional love is the most powerful known stimulant of the immune system" (p. 181).

Just as importantly, this relationship of responsibility lays a heavy obligation on your medical community. I mean a profound insight into the intimate relationship between illness and the ills that afflict our society. For if illness does not occur in a vacuum, then your treatment of illness dare not occur in a vacuum. CEOs and surgeons, internists and nurses, radiologists and anesthesiologists, you will not lead Georgetown into the 21st century if you operate with a tunnel vision, if your administrative ability is bounded by red ink and black, if your surgery reveals simply a superb artist or a journeyman mechanic, if your eyes cannot see beyond the immediate cause of malnutrition or a gunshot wound, a smoke-filled lung or an intestinal inflammation, high blood pressure or rheumatoid arthritis.

Several decades ago I discovered, mainly by reading, that I could not understand my country today if I did not know where America came from and where it's been. The realization complemented an earlier discovery from my specialization in the early church and its theologians: I could not understand my church today if I did not know where it came from and where it's been. Somewhat later I discovered, mainly by looking within, that I could not understand who I am if I did not know where I came from and where I've been. May I suggest that the health care leaders of the 21st century will be the communities that are concerned to discover where their patients come from and where they've been? Not only their medical history in a narrow sense; their broader experience of human and inhuman living; their integral humanity. Our health care leaders will be those who have listened to, have actually heard, the cries of the poor.

In brief, the Jesuit tradition insists that, to be leaders, we must expand the horizons of our health care. Not only more patients to examine and heal. Even more important, an acute awareness of society that shapes so many of these unfortunates and shunts them to our hospitals and mental institutions, to our jails and homes for the unproductive elderly. With that, an uncommon understanding of the bruised images of God you are privileged to serve, understanding their story. Not dividing health care ministry into bodies for doctors and souls for chaplains. A more unified ministry, where all who serve are touching a total person—a person with a story that is intimately related to his or her healing.

C. Preferential Option for Community

The villain in the piece is the rugged individualism Robert Bellah saw conquering American society. I used to think that American Catholicism was not similarly infected—at least that we were less infected. I thought so—until Bellah addressed the Catholic Theological Society some years ago. He mentioned that an obvious counteragent to rugged individualism would seem to be an organization that called itself the Body of Christ, wherein no one could say to any other, "I have no need of you." Regrettably, he concluded, his research reveals that American Catholics are no better in this respect than their non-Catholic sisters and brothers.

The fact is, all who practice medicine are inescapably part and parcel of a community. The medical community is an impressive array of dedicated men and women, vowed to preserve life and prevent death.

You share your knowledge, your expertise, with one another, from the daily rounds to the research into cancer and AIDS. You give freely and free of your time and your talents to so many of the crucified beyond Reservoir Road, from Lorton and Adams Morgan to Latin America and the Far East; eight FAX pages of community service demonstrate this beyond dispute. I am convinced that you have a community that comprises doctor and patient, the nurse and the nursed, the powerful and the powerless, Blue Cross and true cross. But a neuralgic question remains for the next millennium: Is there still a line that has not been crossed? Is the community link a narrowly medical one? Does society distance the healer from the sufferer in subtle but terribly real ways? What do you actually hear when you ask me to cough, to breathe deep, to say "ah?" Do you hear a person? Do you hear the cry of the poor? Do you really hear my story? And if you do, how do you respond?

The Jesuit response, I suggest, takes flesh in a true tale, a story that may serve as a sort of summary of all I have said. A remarkable Hasidic rabbi, Levi Yitzhak of Berdichev in the Ukraine, used to say that he had discovered the meaning of love from a drunken peasant. The rabbi was visiting the owner of a tavern in the Polish countryside. As he walked in, he saw two peasants at a table. Both were gloriously in their cups. Arms around each other, they were protesting how much each loved the other. Suddenly Ivan said to Peter: "Peter, tell me, what hurts me?" Bleary-eyed, Peter looked at Ivan: "How do I know what hurts you?" Ivan's answer was swift: "If you don't know what hurts me, how can you say you love me?"

When all is said and done, when all my research has been completed, when all the arts of rhetoric have dressed it up, the Jesuit tradition in medicine, the Jesuit history of healing, the Jesuit expectation of a doctor or nurse comes down to a short question, five momentous monosyllables from you to me: "Tell me, what hurts you?" Not only the inflamed ileum, the hiatus hernia, the distressing diverticula. Together with all that, what hurts *me*—this unique, unrepeatable person, this commingling of flesh and spirit in the image and likeness of God? Not to have you play psychiatrist, but to rouse the love that may not always cure but has a tremendous capacity to heal.

In four months, God willing, I expect to bear out a sentence of the Hebrew Psalmist: "The days of our life are 70 years, or perhaps 80 if we are strong" (Psalms 90:10). I shall not treasure epithet "octogenarian." What I do treasure are vivid memories (most recently here at Georgetown) of doctors and nurses, administrators and therapists, faculty and students, who made the Jesuit tradition come alive, who not only cured but cared, who not only listened to but actually heard the cries of this state-of-the-art hypochondriac, who in the tradition of Bernie Siegel not only made medicine a practice of joyful love but in the process helped me to love myself more completely.

Notes

[1] See Mary Rose *McGeady* (1991). *God's lost children: Letters from Covenant House.* New York: Covenant House, p. 31.
[2] See Christine Gorman (1993). "When AIDS strikes parents." *Time,* 142, no. 18, Nov. 1, p. 76.
[3] See the editorial (1993). "Children too ready to die young." *Washington Post,* Nov. 3, p. A26.
[4] See *Time,* 128, no. 10, Sept. 8, 1986, p. 57.

References

Bellah, RN (1982). Religion and power in America today. *Commonwealth,* 109 (21) Dec. 3.
Cahill, MD, KM (1991). Introduction. *Imminent peril: Public health in a declining economy.* New York: Twentieth Century Fund.
Catholic Health World (1988). 4 (13) July 1.
C Cepress (ed.). (1993). *Sister Thea Bowman, shooting star: Selected writings and speeches.* Winona, MN: Saint Mary's Press.
McGrath, CSC, M (1986). Social teaching since the Council: A response from Latin America. In A Stacpoole (ed.). *Vatican II revisited by those who were there.* Minneapolis: Winston.
Cuomo, MM (1991). Public health: Old truth, new realities. In KM Cahill, MD (ed.). *Imminent peril: Public health in a declining economy.* New York: Twentieth Century Fund.
Editorial (1993). Children too ready to die young, *Washington Post,* Nov. 3.
Gorman, C (1993). When AIDS strikes parents. *Time,* 142(18).

McGeady, MR (1991). *God's lost children: Letters from Covenant House.* New York: Covenant House.
Siegel, MD, BS (1988). *Love medicine and miracles.* New York: Harper & Row.
Time (1986). 128 (10).

6. Jos V.M. Welie

"For Whom and For What?"
Education and Research in the
Medical and Dental Sciences

I. Introduction

The United States spends a greater part of its national gross product on health care than any other nation. It can boost some of the finest hospitals worldwide and is generally acknowledged to be at the forefront of innovative biomedical research. Indeed, a 2000 World Health Organization (WHO) report on health care systems notes that Americans themselves believe the US system to best respond to the needs of the country when compared to systems elsewhere (WHO, 2000). But the same WHO report also ranks the US health care system 37th in overall performance. This low ranking is due in large part to the unequal distribution of care. Approximately one in seven US citizens still has no health care insurance and approximately twice that many are inadequately insured. Consequently, millions of Americans, including many children, are underserved. This problem of unequal access with its resulting health disparities is not limited to medical care. It also plagues many other domains of health care, in some cases even more painfully than in medicine. For example, more than 108 million children and adults lack dental insurance, which is more than two-and-a-half times the number who lack medical insurance. More than one third of the US population (or some 100 million people) have no access to community water fluoridation, one of the most important components of preventive oral care.

Health economists, administrators and policy makers are acutely aware of the startling (oral) health disparities and many reports have been written of late that address this problem, identifying a variety of activities that will have to be undertaken. An example in point is the 2002 report from the National Institute of Dental and Craniofacial Research entitled *A Plan to Eliminate Health Disparities* (NIDCR, 2002). It advocates scientific research about physiological, genetic and pathological factors that may contribute to the disparities in certain populations, as well as preventive and therapeutic modalities. Psychosocial, legal, administrative and other systemic conditions that cause members of certain populations to become patients in disproportionate numbers must be identified. And financial barriers to the provision of equitable care must be examined and where possible relieved.

There is, however, one factor that most assuredly contributes to health disparities but that is remarkably absent from the discussions. We find listed the many *dental conditions* demanding improved oral care; there are the *patients* who are not adequately cared for; there is the systemic and financial *context* in which care is to be provided. But there is no mention of the *care providers* themselves, the professions of dentistry and dental hygiene. And yet, amelioration, let alone resolution of the problem of oral health care disparities, is intrinsically tied to the willingness and ability of the oral health care providers to share responsibility.

For example, the NIDRC report concludes that there are "striking disparities in dental disease by income. Poor children suffer twice as much dental caries as their more affluent peers and their disease is more likely to be untreated" (NIDCR 2002, Table 1). The passive language in which the report phrases this conclusion suggests that there are no identifiable persons who have failed to treat these children and can be held responsible for the resulting health disparity. These children "are untreated." Yet one could have also phrased the same conclusion in active language: "As a group, dentists and hygienists tend to under treat poor children when compared to their more affluent peers."

Or consider the following observation in the Surgeon General's report, *Oral Health Care in America* (United States Public Health Service, 2000, chapter 4). After pointing out that the caries rate tends to be much higher among adults with disabilities, the report goes on to state that there is also considerable variation among disabled adults, caused in part by where these people reside. If people live in large institutions where services are available, their caries rate is lower when compared to those living in the community "where services must be secured from community practitioners." Although this observation is unusual in its reference to care providers, the diagnosis still is one of disabled patients' failing to secure care from the providers, rather than providers' failing to assure adequate or at least equal, care for disabled patients.

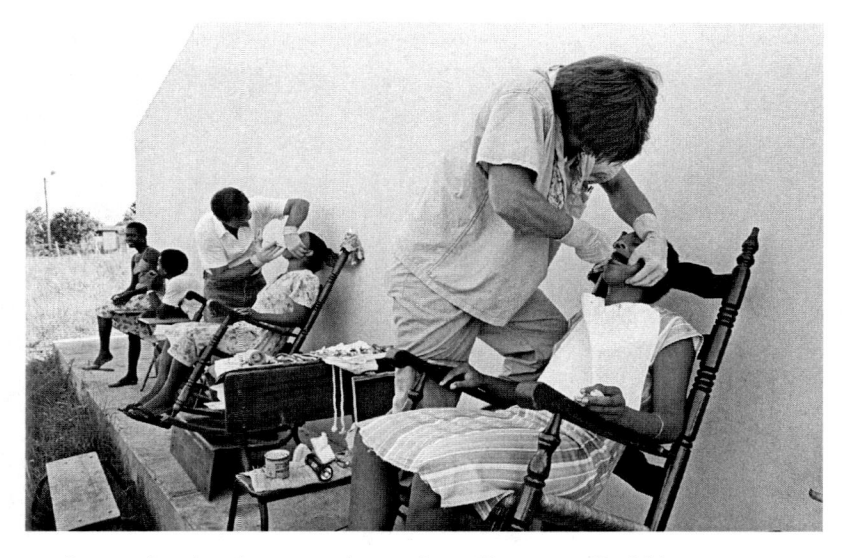

"... are dental students trained to perform effective yet affordable treatments that they can also offer indigent patients once they are in private practice?"
Photographer: Don Doll, SJ

Many other conclusions in these public health reports could likewise be rephrased in active language. The problem is not or at least not only, that there are health disparities, that certain patient populations remain untreated or are under treated. Part of the problem is that oral health care professionals do not treat these patient categories as frequently, consistently and effectively as they treat "mainstream" populations.

This foregoing linguistic critique is not intended to suggest that dentists and hygienists are solely responsible for the existing oral health care. Clearly they are not. However oral health care professionals cannot and may not hide behind the deceptive force of passive language either, as if they carry no responsibility whatsoever for the existing crisis. Precisely as members of the *profession* of oral health care, dentists, dental hygienists and other oral health care providers are called and obligated to address the needs of all patients, including patients who are socially marginalized, indigent, physically or mentally impaired or otherwise at risk of being under treated.

The American Dental Association (ADA) in its *Code of Ethics* specifically states that "dentists have an obligation to use their skills, knowledge and experience for the improvement of the dental health of

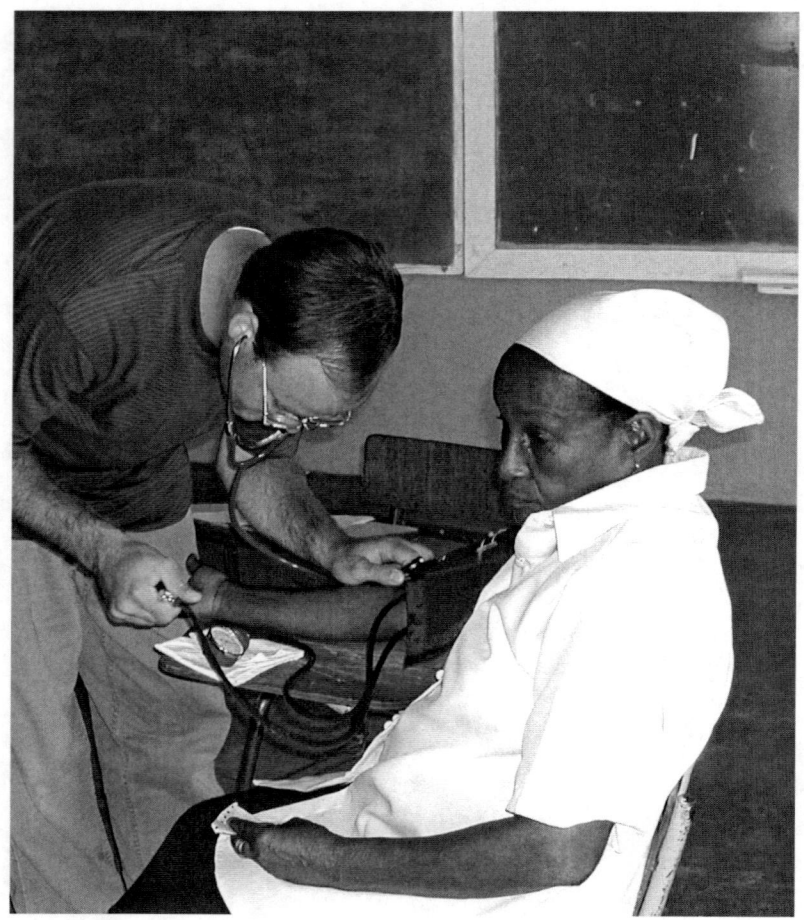

". . . oral health care providers individually and as a profession are called to share in the challenging burden of reducing oral health disparities by providing treatment to the underserved." Photographer: Terry Wilwerding

the *public.*" Moreover, "the dentists' *primary* obligation is service to the patient *and the public-at-large*" (§3—italics added). This obligation also rests on the dental profession at large which must "actively seek allies throughout society on specific activities that will help improve *access to care for all*" (§4—italics added). In its *Ethics Handbook for Dentists*, the American College of Dentists likewise insists that "Dentistry should be available, within reason, to *all* seeking treatment" (ACD, 2000, 8—italics added). These statements underscore that oral health care providers individually and as a profession are called to share in the challenging burden of reducing oral health disparities by providing treatment to the underserved.

It would be unfair to expect a novice swimmer to jump after a person drowning in a deep and muddy lake. Likewise, it would be unfair to expect oral health care professionals to live up to their calling unless they are adequately prepared for this challenge. Dentists must be provided with the education and training necessary to understand and appreciate the predicament of underserved patients. They must learn to discern the particular needs and concerns of diverse categories of underserved patients. They must be taught to correctly diagnose their condition and the factors causing or contributing to the condition. They must be trained to design and implement a treatment plan that is tailored to the needs of these patients, that is effective and satisfactory, yet affordable. The same is true for members of other health professions. This means that a primary role in the struggle against health disparities is to be played by the institutions of higher education that prepare health care professionals.

Any dental school that professes to train dental professionals committed and able to assume the professional challenges outlined by the American Dental Association and the American College of Dentists (as cited above) will have to reexamine whether its curriculum and research agenda adequately prepares its graduates for these tasks. But this is ever the more true of those dental schools that profess to be committed specifically to the poor, marginalized and vulnerable in our society, above all the schools that are sponsored by the Society of Jesus (of which there are three in the US and several more elsewhere in the world).[1] As Massaro has shown in his contribution to this volume, this "preferential option for the poor" was not coined by educators, let alone by Jesuit educators. This maxim was first proposed and contextualized by the Roman Catholic bishops from Latin America at their 1968 conference in Medellin. However, six years later this commitment to "the promotion of justice" was adopted by the 32nd Congregation of the Society of Jesus (1974-75) as a hallmark of the Society and a point of focus in all of its missions, including higher education. More recently, Father Peter-Hans Kolvenbach, the Superior General of the Society, called upon all Jesuit colleges and universities to revisit and where necessary to adjust, their educational, research, service and administrative programs and systems to promote a concern for justice (see his contribution elsewhere in this volume). It is therefore only fitting and fair that we examine whether and how the Jesuit dental and other health sciences schools have transformed their goals, contents and methods to realize this mission call. Indeed, such an examination may be helpful for all health sciences educators and administrators who struggle with the challenging mission of educating health care providers able and ready to tackle the urgent problem of health disparities.

II. Education for Justice in the Health Sciences

In October of 2000, some 400 delegates from the 28 Jesuit colleges and universities in the US convened at Santa Clara University, California's oldest institution of higher education, to discuss the pursuit of social justice as a central theme for Jesuit higher education. This justice-for-education conference followed three years of self-study at each institution, identifying the extent to which the institution had been successful in developing educational programs that educate students to be "men and women for others," concerned about and able to effectively participate in the struggle against social injustice. Kolvenbach reminded the gathered delegates that, "Jesuit universities have stronger and different reasons than many other academic and research institutions for addressing the actual world as it unjustly exists and for helping to reshape in the light of the Gospel." (See his contribution elsewhere in this volume.) He challenged each university and college, each school and program, to revisit all of its teaching,

"For Whom & for What?" Education & Research in Medical & Dental Science 117

research and service missions as well as its processes, systems and structures in light of the Jesuit university's "responsibility for human society that is so scandalously unjust, so complex to understand and so hard to change" (Part IV).

Kolvenbach's reflections, when specifically applied to the context of health sciences education, would suggest that Jesuit health sciences schools are charged to deliver graduates for whom care for the poor and vulnerable is not a matter of optional kindness and charity but a defining aspect of their professional practice. In the words of Pellegrino and Thomasma, "The preferential option for the poor is not simply an 'option' for Christians. It is an obligation to choose to care for the poor to a greater extent than that found in secular society" (1997, 121).

This is not an easy task. It is therefore surprising that the aforementioned national conference at Santa Clara University was attended by relatively few delegates from the Jesuit health sciences schools and programs (approximately a dozen in total). In fact, the self-studies from the various universities, including those with health sciences divisions, reflect this relative absence from the debate. Their absence was ever the more noticeable because other professional schools, specifically business and law, were properly represented and engaged. Why this silence on the part of the health sciences? Several answers can be given to this question, some of which have in fact been given by faculty members and administrators at health sciences schools.

A first answer is that health care, health sciences education and biomedical research, when done well, already realize this justice mission. The greatest service one can do for the marginalized and poor is to simply educate the very best health care providers. This view is advocated by Joan Hrubetz, Dean of St. Louis University School of Nursing, when she writes: "Contemporary nursing with its emphasis on physical, spiritual and emotional health or in other words, the whole person, is uniquely related to the Jesuit mission. Nursing, it has been said, is the Jesuit mission" (1993, p. 18). In other words, the question of what it could mean for a school of nursing to be Jesuit is moot. Running a school of nursing is always consistent with the Jesuit identity of the university at large. Based on my own interviews of several health sciences faculty and administrators at Creighton University, I would suggest that Hrubetz' view is actually widespread. I frequently was told that the provision of health care and hence health sciences education and research, is always for the good of people and thus qualifies as service to God. Hence, health sciences schools at Jesuit universities are always operating in accordance with the institutions' Catholic and Jesuit identity and its mission to foster care for the poor and marginalized.

This is most definitely a comfortable position. Faculty who move from a non-Jesuit health sciences school to a Jesuit one need not make any adjustments and vice versa. Of course, this also means that in times of financial exigency when running health sciences programs is too great a risk for a Jesuit university or even amounts to a financial drain on the university as a whole, it only makes sense to close such programs. If there is no urgent need to invest scarce financial and personnel resources in health sciences programs, one ought not maintain these expensive programs. One may as well leave the instruction of and research in these disciplines to public universities. After all, any good school of nursing is thereby a Jesuit school of nursing, even if it does not profess to be so. Indeed, in the course of the 20th century, at least seven US Jesuit medical, dental and pharmacy schools closed their doors.

A second answer to the question raised above is that Jesuit health sciences education centers, like other non-Jesuit Catholic institutions, have always been and still are, heavily involved in indigent care. In so doing, they aptly fulfill their Jesuit educational mission. It is most assuredly correct that the faculty and students at the clinics of Jesuit universities treat many indigent and marginalized patients who cannot afford to obtain care elsewhere. But the question remains whether this service to the poor constitutes so-called "service learning" as well. Of course, students always learn from their engagement in worthy social causes. They may gain awareness of and concern for the less fortunate in our society. But such learning does not qualify as education proper as it is typically offered by institutions of higher education. That is to say, one does not have to be a student at a (Jesuit) university to gain that kind of learning. Anybody who engages in these worthy social causes will gain the same learning. It is only when such service activities are offered as a logical part of a structured course with specified objectives, teaching method and measurable outcomes that they qualify as educational activities.

If we grant this, then it is not at all clear that the health sciences students who treat indigent and other marginalized patients typically do so in the context of a structured course that specifically focuses on the problems of indigent and marginalized patients. In fact, I venture to guess that generally this is not the case. These poor and marginalized patients are simply added to the pool of patients to be treated. At times, the supervising instructor may challenge the student to consider the impact of the patient's social marginalization on her medical condition. Or the patient's inability to pay for the recommended dental treatment may force the student to think in terms of basic care that is affordable. But these experiences are seldom part of a course that is specifically targeted to health care needs of indigent or otherwise underserved patient populations.

Paradoxically, this lack of a structural embedding of the health care rendered to the poor may have two undesirable consequences. First, the graduates may believe that they have done their share of charitable care by the time they leave the institution. This unfortunate outcome is fostered if the students, who are already paying in excess of $30,000 tuition annually, are expected to pay for the treatments when patients fail to do so lest they lose the educational credit for the treatments performed. Second, students and even more so faculty and administrators, may lose sight of the fact that the poor and vulnerable are not just recipients of care; they also serve as objects of learning and research. Throughout modern history, the poor and vulnerable have borne a disproportionate share of the burden as objects of medical teaching and research. This ought to render us cautious in too quickly describing our care for indigent and vulnerable populations as our altruistic contribution toward justice.

Even if genuine service learning programs are added to the existing health sciences curricula, sensitizing students to the needs of the poor and vulnerable, and increasing their understanding of the prevalence, causes and consequences of these social injustices, the question remains whether the scientific and technical training they receive allows them to optimally address the needs of the poor. For example, are dental students trained to perform effective yet affordable treatments that they can also offer indigent patients once they are in private practice? Or are they trained foremost to perform high-end dental procedures that their indigent patients can only afford because the school has substantially discounted the fees in order to attract patients? Yet once these students have become independent dentists, the same patients no longer can get the same treatment from the same dentists because the latter have to charge far more than the patients can afford?

The third answer to our question why it is that the Jesuit health sciences schools have not been equally engaged in the education-for-justice project, is directly tied to the issue identified in the former paragraph. Even if the Jesuit health sciences schools would want to create educational programs that train health care professionals to make a real difference for the many poor and vulnerable patients, they simply cannot do so. The standardization of health sciences education that has come about through accreditation and licensing examinations forces Jesuit health sciences schools to closely match the curricula at their non-Jesuit counterparts, of which there are after all far more.

This is most certainly a genuine concern. There is no point in educating health care professionals who, upon graduation, cannot obtain a license to practice. But there is probably more latitude than may appear at first sight. The close match between Jesuit health sciences programs and their non-Jesuit counterparts in many an instance may be intentional rather than the result of enforced standards. After all, these Jesuit health sciences schools are all private schools and hence receive no (or relatively little) state support. Their survival hinges on the number of students they attract. Even a small decrease could prove to be fiscally fatal. Few administrators therefore will be eager to risk their neck by adopting a counter-cultural curriculum if this could result in a decrease of their student applicant pool. Some years ago I asked a senior administrator from my own medical school in what regard the curriculum at our Catholic and Jesuit school differed from the curricula at the many secular medical schools in the country. Clearly surprised by my question, the administrator answered that our curriculum had been explicitly designed *not* to differ from that of other medical schools.

The same is true for the area of biomedical research. Scientific programs heavily rely on the subsidies and grants from the medical and pharmaceutical industries. These companies are not primarily interested in the health care needs of the indigent and marginalized in society. They are not the ones who spend fourteen per cent of the national gross product on health care goods and services. Even public funding for biomedical research (as it is available through the National Institutes of Health) is impacted by powerful lobbies, few of which represent society's poor and marginalized.

These are all valid concerns and they may pose restraints on what Jesuit health sciences schools can do with their curricula and research agendas. If a society—for example, as a result of its strict separation of church and state and the resulting limitations on the allocation of tax income; or through its educational standards and research priorities—renders it *de facto* impossible for the Society of Jesuit to sponsor an academic medical center, so be it. Nobody, not even the Society of Jesus, is morally required to do what cannot be done. But in that case, these schools should either close their doors or continue their otherwise excellent work in higher education as secular schools.

But then again, the question remains whether the situation is as grim as it may appear at first sight. Consider for example the availability of public funding for dental research. The National Institutes of Health has launched several major funding opportunities to reduce health disparities. Similar funds are available through large private organizations such as the Robert Wood Johnson Foundation. This is but one example that suggests that where there is a will there is a way. Instead of competing for students with the rich and famous among the nation's medical schools and health sciences centers, one could also "build the field" and trust that the students and the necessary dollars will come. After all, what financial guarantees did Ignatius of Loyola (1491-1556) have when he established the first Jesuit colleges and universities, more than 30 of them in the last eight years of his life? That feat is ever the more remarkable since he prohibited the schools from charging any tuition at all.

III. The Historical Origins of Jesuit Health Sciences

An interesting "detail" in the history of Jesuit education is that Ignatius determined that the universities sponsored by the Society would not include faculties of medicine or law, deeming these disciplines "more remote" to the educational mission of the Society. There is ample evidence that this constitutional exclusion of medical schools did not reflect Ignatius' views on the importance of health and health care, for he clearly favored these goods (or at least came to favor them in the latter part of his life (Welie; 2003a). A more likely explanation of the exclusion is that Ignatius saw no need to devote scarce personnel resources to the instruction of medical sciences (or law). Secular universities were already doing a fine job in these areas. The real needs lay in the area of theological education (and the prerequisites for a study in theology (Welie 2003b). This would also explain why the constitutional exclusion was not absolute. Medical and law schools could be incorporated into Jesuit universities provided this would not require Jesuits to administer them or teach the courses. Indeed, the Jesuit university at Pont-à-Mousson (France) was the first to include a medical school, but its dean and professors were all lay. Once established in the early 17th century, the medical school became popular and successful. However, the institution withered after the city of Pont-à-Mousson was overtaken by King Louis XIII, until it was finally transferred to the nearby city of Nancy in 1768 (Ganss, 1969). Shortly thereafter, the Society was suppressed and all the Jesuit schools were closed.

There is some similarity between this early history of Jesuit health sciences education in the Old World and the developments in the New World. Of the 28 Jesuit universities in the US, fewer than a quarter once had medical schools and that number is now down to four.[2] Only three still have a dental school (down from six)[3] and one a school of pharmacy (down from three).[4] The question thus remains whether health sciences education still is "more remote" to the educational mission of the Society. When at the dawn of the 21st century, Ignatius' 29th successor Father Kolvenbach, admonished representatives of the 28 US Jesuit colleges and universities gathered at Santa Clara University to promote justice by serving the poor, did he first and foremost address the faculties in the programs of theology, humanities, arts and sciences, and business or also those in the more than 50 remaining health sciences degree programs in the US alone?

Ignatius insisted that his fellow Jesuits care for the hospitalized. Most assuredly he would do the same today if it weren't for the fact that the hospitalized of today are not the same as the hospitalized of the mid-16th century. The hospitals in Ignatius' day and age simply cannot be compared with a 21st century hospital. Medieval hospitals were places where the poor, the sick and the marginalized could find shelter, a bed, food and some basic care. They were more akin to modern homeless shelters. The question thus arises whether Ignatius, upon visiting a 21st century academic medical center, would still find that it realizes the objectives of the Society in a clear and convincing manner, worthy of the large investments by his Society.

Superior General Peter-Hans Kolvenbach has pointed out that "Ignatius stressed the education of future 'doctores' as the practical end of a Jesuit university." But even if "higher education as both means and medium has intrinsic value, it must still always ask itself: 'For whom? For what?' The answer to these questions will always be related to the common good and the progress of human society" (Kolvenbach, 2001, §26). Reflecting on his days as provincial in the Middle East, he notes:

> In Beirut we were well aware that our medical school, staffed by very holy Jesuits, was producing, at least at that time, some of the most corrupt citizens in the city, but this was taken for granted. The social mood of the explosive Near East did not favor a struggle against sinful, unjust structures. . . . The Christian churches had committed themselves to many works of charity, but involvement in the promotion of justice would have tainted them by association with leftist movements and political turmoil (see Kolvenbach's contribution elsewhere in this volume).

For whom and for what are we presently training health care professionals? Are we educating professionals who are both committed to the care of the poor and marginalized and sufficiently knowledgeable and skilled to effectively address their medical needs?

IV. Contemporary Health Sciences Education for Justice

As the last question makes clear, I am assuming that clinicians, precisely as clinicians, are both charged and able to care for the poor and vulnerable. Granted, there are multiple systemic and structural causes to the grave injustices in the world of health care that defy the efforts of the individual clinician qua clinician. Clinicians should be educated about these systemic and structural factors so as to become informed advocates for change. A health sciences curriculum for justice hence must contain courses on the health care system, economics and policy development. But such advocacy does not qualify as clinical care proper. Most graduates from Jesuit health sciences schools will become clinicians rather than policy makers. They are charged to promote justice in their own sphere of influence and it is for that work that Jesuit health sciences schools must prepare them adequately.

In what manner can the individual clinician contribute to more justice in health care? Who are the vulnerable and marginalized in the modern world that tend to be neglected by the health care system at large as well as by individual caregivers? We can distinguish two main categories of vulnerable patients.

There are those who by virtue of social, economic or other non-medical factors become vulnerable. Their medical symptoms and conditions may not differ from those of patients in general, but because of these non-medical factors they are unable to reach the health care system, communicate with caregivers or afford the care they need. In order to address these needs, we must train health care providers to provide basic care, wherein the term "basic" has multiple connotations: basic as in low-tech; basic as in comprehensible; basic as in affordable; basic as in universal.

The second category of vulnerable patients are those whose very medical condition causes them to be at risk for medical neglect. This is because the medical system tends to focus on certain diseases, treatment modalities and categories of patients while paying relatively little attention to others. There are many reasons for this "favoritism" and it tends to vary by historical period and country. At present, it would seem that western medicine tends to focus on acute medical needs, curative care, interventions that are technologically advanced and elective treatments that are commercially profitable. Consequently, patients with terminal illnesses that demand a palliative approach tend to be marginalized. So are mentally disabled patients, elderly with chronic illnesses and children in need of preventive care.

If Jesuit-trained physicians, dentists, nurses and other health care professionals are to give a preferential option to these "poor" and relieve their needs, it is up to Jesuit educational institutions to adequately prepare them for this task. This means that the curricula of the various health sciences degree programs must provide students with the necessary theoretical and practical training. A Jesuit physical therapy program can only expect its graduates to treat indigent patients if it has taught them how to provide sound physical therapy care with a modest investment of material resources and time, thus keeping the charges to the patients down yet generating sufficient income to the therapist. A Jesuit medical school can only expect its graduates to provide optimal end-of-life care if it has provided them with the latest expertise in pain treatment as well as the necessary legal knowledge to feel comfortable prescribing narcotic drugs. A dental school can only expect its graduates to care for patients with advanced Alzheimer's dementia if it has familiarized students with this disease, its symptoms, the patients who suffer from it and the nursing homes where they live.

It is not easy to determine what curricular changes need to be executed in order to make sure that graduates from Jesuit health sciences degree programs have a thorough understanding of the plight of the underserved; are motivated to improve their plight not only as fellow-citizens and as societal leaders but also, and precisely, as health care providers; and are competent to effectively and efficiently provide the needed health care to those patients. In each disciplinary area, research must be undertaken to pinpoint exactly the connections between inequalities in clinical care rendered and the existing curriculum; to determine what additions to the curriculum may improve the education of our students; to develop instructional methods that effectively achieve these learning objectives; and if necessary even to change the overall culture in the school.

Lacking familiarity with the scope and nature of the most health sciences degree programs and the contents of their respective curricula, I am not able even to speculate about the specific curricular adjustments that would have to be made in each of these programs. I therefore limit myself to some tentative examples from two degree programs with which I am somewhat more familiar, that is, medicine and dentistry. Pending a scientifically supported proposal, I submit that the curriculum at a Jesuit medical school that professes to educate physicians who will be ready and able to care for the most vulnerable patients in our modern society will contain a disproportionate—that is, in comparison to non-Jesuit schools—number of credit hours in such disciplines as public health and preventive medicine, perinatal medicine, family practice, geriatrics, psychiatry and mental health care, palliative medicine and terminal care. A dental curriculum for justice likewise would place heavy emphasis on preventive and community dentistry, basic dental care, dental care for patients with mental or physical disabilities, geriatric dentistry and nursing home oral health care. The courses in these disciplines, in addition to regular scientific and technical training, should be further enriched with service learning projects.

Evidently, it would not be possible to simply expand the time allotted to the aforementioned subjects without cutting into the curriculum elsewhere. Most health sciences curricula are already overfilled, leaving students little time to engage in extracurricular formation activities or even with their families. This condition of permanent stress does not favor an attitude of concern for the least among us (see also Stempsey's contribution elsewhere in this volume). But as soon as we begin to list disciplinary areas that are to be sacrificed in order to make time for justice-related subjects, the suggestion is made that those disciplines fail to contribute to more justice in health care; or, even worse, they counteract justice.

The suggestion that certain health sciences courses could counteract justice is most certainly false. All of health care can contribute to the care of the poor and vulnerable in society and when properly applied, no health care causes injustice. No specialty disqualifies its practitioners of service for the poor and vulnerable. Even esthetic surgery and dentistry, though increasingly used to cater to the vanity of patients who have money to spare, can also be practiced in the service of those whose deformities, traumas or tattoos have rendered them socially vulnerable. In fact, this discussion is not about the disciplines themselves but about the patient populations on which they tend (not) to focus. It is about shifting emphases. Instead of focusing on the health care needs of people who have a voice and are already being listened to by the hundreds of medical, dental and other non-Jesuit health sciences degree programs in the United States alone, the Jesuit health sciences schools and programs must listen to the silent outcries of the voiceless in society.

V. Concluding Reflections

"The preferential option for the poor is not simply an 'option' for Christians. It is an obligation to choose to care for the poor to a greater extent than that found in secular society." In their 1997 book, *Helping and Healing: Religious Commitment in Health Care,* Pellegrino and Thomasma have outlined how the option for the poor not only applies to the design of health care systems and national debates about allocation of scarce resources, but also to "admission criteria to medical schools" (156). In this chapter, I have argued that even the latter does not suffice. For example, an increase in the number of minority students at a medical school does not guarantee that these students, upon graduation will be motivated and capable of providing health care to underserved populations. In order for that to happen, the very curriculum and research agenda of the institution must be imbued with a concern for the vulnerable and marginalized in society.

History is full of stories about poor patients receiving poor treatment from poor doctors—that is to say, about socially marginalized patients receiving grossly inadequate treatment from callous or incompetent doctors. At the dawn of the 21st century, the marginalized patients are still with us, even in a wealthy nation such as the United States. Many still receive inadequate treatment. In part, this problem is caused by a failing health care system. But the system is not the only cause. There appears to be a widening gap between new medical treatments developed and their accessibility for all patients such that ever more sophisticated treatments are available for ever fewer patients. And unfortunately, there is still a dearth of competent clinicians motivated and capable to care for the marginalized and vulnerable in our society.

This situation of inequality is not necessarily immoral. From the perspective of free market capitalism, the existing health disparities are unfortunate but not unjust. However, that argument cannot be invoked by any institution professing to operate from a Christian perspective.

> The Christian vocation is quite specifically oriented to a charitable redress of the inequities of nature or circumstance. It is, in fact, precisely to the losers in the natural lottery—the sick, the poor, the outcast—that Christ addressed his personal ministry and his Sermon on the Mount. This is the basis for the preferential option for the poor that inspires the best Christian institutions (Pellegrino & Thomasma, 1997, p. 155).

Acknowledgment

The research supporting this chapter has been made possible in part by a grant from the National Institute of Dental and Craniofacial Research (NIDCR) on the "Impact of Education on Oral Health Disparities" (1 R21 DE014969-01).

Notes

[1] Creighton University in Omaha, Nebraska; University of Detroit-Mercy in Detroit, Michigan; and Marquette University in Milwaukee, Wisconsin.

[2] Creighton, Fordham, Georgetown, Loyola Chicago, Marquette and St. Louis Universities. Fordham and Marquette later closed their medical schools.

[3] Creighton, Detroit-Mercy, Georgetown, Loyola Chicago, Marquette and St. Louis Universities. Georgetown and Loyola closed their dental schools; St. Louis changed its dental school into a postgraduate speciality program for orthodontics. According to Harney (1962, p. 439), there once was a seventh dental school but he does not specify at which Jesuit university.

[4] Creighton University is the only US based Jesuit university with a school of pharmacy. According to Harney (1962, p. 439), there once were three Jesuit schools of pharmacy but he does not specify where.

References

American College of Dentists (ACD) (2000). *Ethics handbook for dentists.* Gaithersburg: ACD. http://www.facd.org/acdethics.htm#EthicsHandbook (site accessed on 7-14-04).

Ganss, GE (1969). *The Jesuit educational tradition and Saint Louis University.* St. Louis: St. Louis University Press.

Harney, MP (1962). *The Jesuit in history. The Society of Jesus through four centuries.* Chicago: Loyola University Press

Hrubetz, J (1993). Nursing education in Jesuit universities and colleges. The art of science and caring. *Conversations,* Spring, 18-19.

Kolvenbach, HP (2001). The Jesuit university in the light of the Ignatian charism. Address at the International Meeting of Jesuit Higher Education, Rome (Monte Cucco), May 27, 2001. http://www.sjweb.info/documents/doc_show.cfm?PubTextId=1607 (site accessed on 7-14-04).

National Institute of Dental and Craniofacial Research (NIDCR) (2002) A plan to eliminate health disparities. Washington, DC: NIDCR. www.nidcr.nih/gov/research/health_disp.asp (site accessed on 7-14-04).

Pellegrino, ED & Thomasma, DC (1997). *Helping and healing: Religious commitment in health care.* Washington DC: Georgetown University Press.

US Public Health Service (2000). *Oral health in America: A report of the Surgeon General.* Washington DC. http://www.nidcr.nih.gov/sgr/oralhealth.asp (site accessed on 7-14-04).

Welie, JVM (2003a). Saint Ignatius' attitude towards the body, health and health care. *National Catholic Bioethics Quarterly,* 3(2) 247-255.

———. (2003b). Ignatius of Loyola on medical education. Or should today's Jesuits continue to run health sciences schools? *Early Science and Medicine,* 8(1) 26-43.

World Health Organization (WHO) (2000). *World health report 2000. Health systems: improving performance.* Geneva: World Health Organization. http://www.who.int/whr2001/2001/archives/2000/en/contents.htm (site accessed on 7-14-04).

7. William E. Stempsey, SJ

Forming Physicians for the Poor: The Role of Medical & Premedical Education

I. Introduction

A man having a severe heart attack was turned away from the downtown clinic of a major health maintenance organization because he was not a member. The receptionist did confer with a nurse, but the nurse refused to come to the lobby to see the man. The receptionist gave him directions to a nearby hospital and he drove himself there, getting lost along the way. Doctors determined that he had ruptured a heart valve and that the resulting blood clots had blocked a coronary artery. The man was transferred to the university hospital where he received intensive therapy and was eventually discharged. Although the clinic fired the two employees involved, stating that their response was "directly contrary" to the clinic's policy of providing emergency medical assistance to any person who needs it (Griffin, 1996), the story illustrates a bureaucratic mind set in today's medicine.

This man had health insurance. His denial of care resulted from a human failure to follow an institutional policy that would have helped him. But in this era of ever-increasing commercialization of health care, things are even worse for the many who do not have any health insurance. While a few strident free-market advocates and those who are just hardhearted maintain that people who cannot afford adequate health care are merely unfortunate and have no claim on the rest of society, the rest of us seem to be at a loss about how to reform the health care system in order to provide adequate care for the most needy.

Sociological and economic analyses are necessary for addressing this problem, but in this chapter I want to go in a different direction—a direction that I believe is equally or even more important.

My claim is that the education of our medical students needs to help them to develop a too-often-ignored dimension of medical care—a social conscience in which the preferential option for the poor plays a central role.

When asked why they want to be doctors, prospective medical students will almost always say that they like science and that they want to help people. These two aspects represent the science and art that have long been taken as the two essential components of medical practice. While it may be more difficult to teach the art of medicine than its science, medical schools have never neglected the teaching of the art.

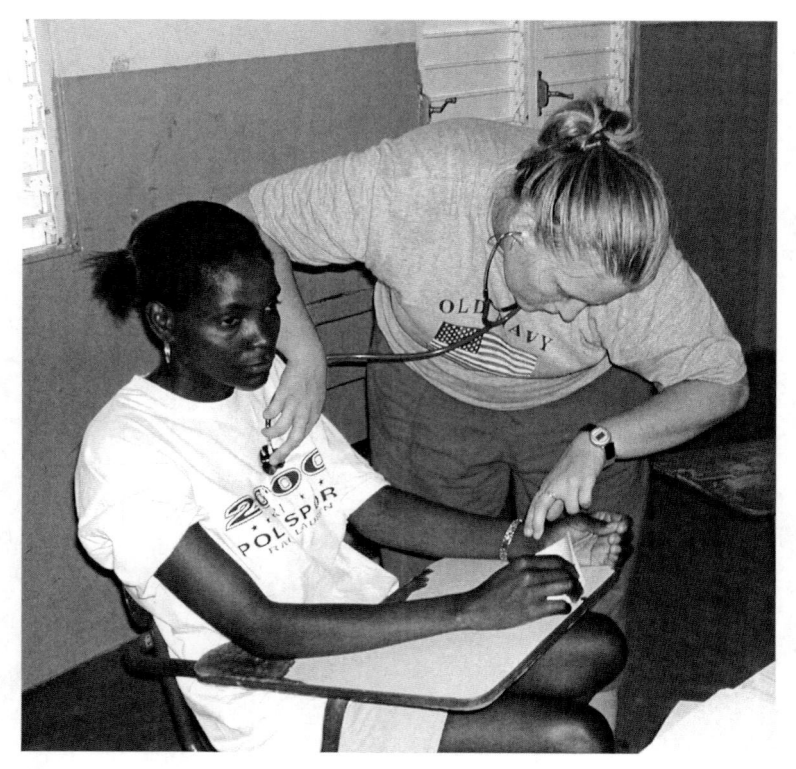

"My claim is that the education of our medical students needs to help them to develop a too-often-ignored dimension of medical care—a social conscience in which the preferential option for the poor plays a central role."
Photographer: Terry Wilwerding

Medical education has always taken the development of humane care-givers as essential to its mission. There is a large literature concerned with the physician-patient relationship and with "humanizing" medicine. But in a society characterized by an increasing gap between the haves and the have-nots, educating physicians to be only technically competent and humane to their patients is not enough. Physicians must also develop a social conscience.

It would be simplistic merely to condemn the commercialization of medicine and to root in this commercialism the loss of altruism among the current crop of students. Money is not the root of this evil; doctors received money for their services long before the advent of managed care and even before the era of indemnity insurance. The real root of the evil is lack of money for those who most need care. A social conscience is as necessary in a government-sponsored health care system as it is in a for-profit hospital.

What I want to suggest is that the preferential option for the poor is a particularly useful way of making specific what a social conscience would entail. In particular, my claim is that a morally adequate system of medical care will not come only from a radical economic restructuring of our health care system (which, in any case, seems unlikely). What is needed is a more fundamental change of attitude. What is needed is for physicians to feel so strongly about caring for the most needy that they will do it! If such attitudes could be fostered, systemic and economic changes will follow.

II. The Problem: Changing Attitudes

Albert Jonsen (1983, p. 1532) points out that a profound moral paradox pervades medicine; this paradox arises from "the incessant conflict of the two most basic principles of morality: self-interest and altruism." This conflict is present everywhere in human life, but according to Jonsen, is inherent in the very structure of medical care. His "moral archeology" unearths two traditions on which modern medical morality is based and from which the conflict arises. One is the ancient Greek literature of the Hippocratic physician whose morals show "precious little altruism" but rather an ethic consisting of "counsels of self-interest." There is nothing inherently unethical about this attitude, especially when seen in the light of the Hippocratic precept that has come to be formulated as *primum non nocere*, but it is not a sufficient moral basis for medicine. It was not until the second century AD that Stoic and Christian influences brought the idea of altruism into the medical literature. The Christian church came to see the care of the sick as a duty of charity (Jonsen, 1983, p. 1533).

According to Jonsen, medical education encourages the paradox between altruism and self-interest. Students come to medical school with mixed motives. They want to earn a good living in a prestigious profession and also be of service to others. But the intense competition for admission to medical school and good residency programs encourages self-interest. At the same time, ceremonial occasions emphasize altruistic ideals. More concretely, the "absolute asceticism of the residency" recreates for physicians-in-training "the sacrificial ethic of monastic medicine." Residency training is severe and fashions for the new physician a conscience that "will ever cry out when self-interest intrudes on patient care" (Jonsen, 1983, p. 1534). It is not easy to envision how medical education could remove this paradox, but it might be able to do a much better job in making the paradox explicit. The challenge is to make medical education itself more "sensitive to the way in which it aggravates the paradox" and to make the paradox clear to both physicians and the public in such a way that an honest acknowledgment of it would be of benefit for all (Jonsen, 1983, p. 1535). Raising awareness of the paradox could raise sensitivity to the plight of the poor. Providing care to those who cannot provide remuneration requires that physicians confront the paradox.

The most senior of our physicians point out that attitudes toward caring for the poor have changed substantially over the years. One physician who received his training in the 1920s argues that the physicians who practiced in teaching hospitals were motivated by a grand tradition in medicine: the "gift of care for the poor or disabled" that was "in the highest tradition of altruism" (Graef, 1977, p. 1455). He maintains that altruism in medicine has declined since those days and points to the more recent primacy of physicians' business associations, third-party payment for medical care and changing systems of reimbursement. Many of the municipal hospitals that provided care for the poor in the past also paid residents next to nothing, but they were nonetheless among the most sought-after sites for residency training. Indeed, after World War I the private urban teaching hospitals usually reserved 60 to 80 percent of their beds for free care; a few served almost exclusively charity cases (Ludmerer, 1999, pp. 118-119). By the 1960s, however, this percentage dropped substantially, as free care began to impose a greater and greater financial burden on the hospitals (Ludmerer, 1999, 167, 264-265).

All this sounds hopelessly quaint in the current context of managed care, and it is tempting to see it as the pining of an old man for a Golden Age that may never have actually existed. Such a facile dismissal is too hasty, however, for this old physician's questions might prompt us toward a new way of thinking about what the preferential option for the poor might mean in the contemporary medical context.

Graef (1977, p. 1455) asks: "Should a patient's bill be larger in a teaching hospital? Or should the cost of training be paid for out of general tax revenues?" Today's context makes these questions sound out-of-date and simplistic, but regardless of the changed details of our context, the big question remains. How should society pay for medical training and medical care for the poor? If we are to take seriously the preferential option for the poor, what does justice demand?

Graef maintains that young physicians (those who were young in the late 1970s) are no different from their counterparts in other professions with respect to the pressures to maximize skills and income and to provide for family. What is in danger of being lost, however, is the "priceless heritage to serve regardless of financial reward" (Graef, pp.1977 & 1455). It is here that the connection between altruism, care for the poor and financial structures becomes evident. The challenge—and it is a far more complex challenge today than it was in Graef's day—is to find a way to make our financial schemes serve our altruism rather than trying to tailor our altruism to fit our financial plans. Fostering an altruistic attitude must take priority. If physicians and society are truly committed in this way, the financial plan that will foster these ideals will follow.

An oral history project at the Yale University School of Medicine, carried out in the late 1970s and early 1980s, gives some interesting insight into medical students' attitudes about serving the poor. The ethos of many of the more prestigious medical school is research-oriented. Once again, the message of the primacy of science is transmitted. This orientation subtly discourages students from the primary care careers that would be of most service to the poor. One student interested in primary care put it this way:

> The ethic of the school is not to encourage students to enter any of the primary care fields. And this is to be expected. At least ninety percent of my classmates intend to go into subspecialty or academic medicine. . . . I guess I've come to realize that illness stems from many causes, some biological, some social, some behavioral. It's not easy to approach a sick patient with only one model in mind. Primary care gives me the best opportunity to combine all these elements (Viseltear, 1985, p. 41).

Role models are crucial in all education and interns and residents are the primary role models for medical students in their clinical years. Some students are appalled at the attitudes they find in house staff. Some are even adamant about changing the attitudes of their peers. One black medical student noted that a resident continually referred to one particular patient as "dumb." The student said:

> She could have been any of a hundred people I knew growing up in New York City and I couldn't explain my feelings because we were simply on different wavelengths. He's never seen a ghetto or an alcoholic or a drug addict. And neither have eighty percent of my class. Perhaps that's why I chose Yale. Perhaps my sensitivity will rub off on some of my fellow students (Viseltear, 1985, pp. 45-46).

Another black student, seeing the need to go beyond sensitivity training, explicitly talked about social concerns for the poor and the importance of physicians in fostering social change.

> Look, what I'm suggesting is nothing that others haven't already said better and louder hundreds of times before. The problem is that the same issues championed a decade ago are still with us today. Now we've come to realize that many of these issues cut across different boundaries and affect various constituencies. It's not just blacks who are concerned here. It's also Hispanics, the elderly, and the poor. All

of us should be concerned and want to do something. It's probably too late, but as future leaders of our nation we better stand up and be counted. You see, everyone, and black people especially, look up to physicians. We're professionals, healers, the valued and respected members of the community. You don't have to be a politician to change society. There's a great deal I can do just by being here and by being myself (Viseltear, 1985, p. 47).

It is a constant wonder to me that so many good and caring physicians emerge from a dehumanizing system of medical education. But the altruism of some students does survive medical training. A few even go beyond being humane and develop the sort of social conscience I am advocating.

> I'm going to make things different if it kills me. I'll get my degree and with it credibility. I'll be in a good social medicine residency program and then fulfill my commitment to the [National Health Service] Corps. And I'll work in a clinic and do family medicine, and perhaps run for a municipal or state office. Or I'll get a job in a federal agency. You see, things have to change. We have to do away with racism. We have to get away from the profit motive. We have to make people care. We have to make government honest and concerned with suffering and need. We have to make our physicians into something other than capitalists interested only in creature comforts (Viseltear, 1985, p. 47).

Such committed students, unfortunately, are a minority. It is too easy for the many to praise the few who serve the poor but have no personal investment in serving the needy themselves. Ginzberg and Brann (1980) taught a course on medicine and society at Columbia University in 1978 and reported on the essays they received from the medical students in their course. Only a minority of students held that health care is a right. Not one student mentioned a desire to practice in a rural setting or in an inner city, citing isolation from medical developments, high crime rates, poor facilities, the absence of career opportunities and the lack of social or intellectual stimulation. Although a few favored "mandatory service programs" to meet national needs, the majority preferred improved incentives for physicians to work in underserved areas. Incentive programs, however, allow the most well-off medical students to ignore the problems of the poor.

Medical education unintentionally leads students away from developing an attitude favorable to serving the poor. Even courses in medical ethics may not help. Sidney Dean Watson (1996) argues that bioethicists have not given proper attention to service to the poor. He admits that bioethics has carefully considered issues of social justice and allocation of resources, but argues that these issues are usually considered at the macro level and not as a matter for individual moral judgment. According to Watson, this is because bioethics has focused its discussions around case studies of interactions between physicians and patients. The problem is that many poor people just do not get any care. When there is no patient, there is no doctor-patient relationship and hence no story to tell. The irony is that virtually all medical students and house staff treat poor people, but the message they receive from their mentors is that "the poor are undesirable and less-deserving of care than others." Medical students "are being taught by example to avoid the poor" (Watson, 1996, p. 363).

If they are trained in private university hospitals, students may actually learn that it is appropriate to turn away the poor. Steven Miles (1992) relates the story of a woman with a fractured arm who was refused treatment at a private not-for-profit university hospital because she had no health insurance. A male acquaintance had assaulted her and after the assault she impulsively took an overdose of an anticonvulsant drug. A friend brought her to the hospital where she was medically stabilized. An orthopedic surgeon determined that her arm required internal fixation to set the fracture. But he declined to take her to surgery because she did not have medical insurance. The woman secretly left the hospital with a central venous catheter in place and went to the county hospital for treatment. The university hospital had treated the woman's life-threatening condition and so it did nothing illegal even though it failed to take care of her broken arm!

Miles argues that these kinds of cases are often presented as anecdotes that illustrate the need for reform of the health care delivery system, but that another perspective on the case is less noticed. This kind of case, which involved a second-year resident, an intern and two medical students, has four adverse consequences for "the next generation of physicians." First, it disrupts the transmission of the "professional tradition that recognized the claim of indigent ill persons on the medical profession." Second, teaching young physicians and their patients that physicians may properly put their own financial interests ahead of their patients' needs breeds cynicism in both doctor and patient. Third, it undermines the ancient message of medical altruism—that physicians are bound by "professing" *humanitas* and *misericordia* to those in need. Fourth, it diminishes physicians' credibility in social debate about health care (Miles, 1992, pp. 2561-2562). Actions speak louder than lectures on ethics and humanism.

This neglect of the poor is usually not malicious. David Hilfiker (1987) relates a story of a homeless man whose jaw had been broken and was wired shut to heal. He was treated properly but discharged from the hospital to return to living on the streets of Washington, D.C. Not surprisingly, he was unable to eat or drink enough to sustain himself and the police found him dehydrated, unconscious and close to death. The physicians who had treated him compassionately just did not understand what life on the streets and in the shelters is like. They had no other option than to discharge this man and they "hardened themselves to the reality of Mr. W.'s plight and talked about discharge to a shelter as if that were a legitimate plan for a demented old man who needed constant supervision" (Hilfiker, 1987, 3155).

Hilfiker realizes how difficult it is to care for such patients. Doing so opens us to the "pain, suffering and, vulnerability of the poor." It forces us to confront our own limitations and the limitations of a society that "refuses to accept responsibility for its broken ones." It is most tempting to turn such patients away, "sparing ourselves the deep frustration." But Hilfiker offers us a challenge.

> I am beginning to realize that we in medicine need the poor to bring us back to our roots as a servant profession. Medicine drifts understandably yet ominously toward the technical and the economically lucrative, and we find it difficult to resist. Perhaps we *need* the poor at this very moment to bring us back to ourselves. The nature of the healer's work is to be with the wounded in their suffering. Can the poor in their very vulnerability show us how (Hilfiker, 1987, p. 3156)?

This is unlikely to make sense to the student narrowly focused on scientific medicine. Yet, allowing the poor to teach what it is like to suffer provides an education in character that no interaction with a professor can provide.

There is a tendency for reports of the many health afflictions of the homeless and the poor tend to "depress and demoralize" us and to make us feel that nothing can be done in the face of such huge problems (Hilfiker, 1989). There is, however, something that can be done. Hilfiker reminds us that the health problems of the poor are associated with other social problems, especially the lack of adequate housing. Physicians could be a potent political force to assure that adequate public funds are allocated to remedy this situation. But how could physicians be persuaded to do this? I would argue that we must select medical students with the promise of developing such a social conscience and that we must help them to develop such attitudes throughout their medical education.

III. Premedical Education and Medical School Admissions

In his American Medical Association (AMA) Presidential Inaugural Address, Alan Nelson (1989) notes that an AMA public opinion survey indicated that fewer than half of Americans feel that doctors explain things well to their patients. Fewer than three in ten think that doctors spend enough time with their patients and more than half think that doctors are too interested in making money. He argues that altruism is an intrinsic part of medical practice that calls for diligence and faithfulness during the times when physicians might be tempted to abandon their patients, whether from fear of contracting an infectious disease or from a desire to avoid those patients who are inconvenient and unprofitable. Unfortunately, compassion often gets lost in the process of learning science. Nelson endorses a broad premedical education in the humanities to foster an altruistic character.

Ouzts and Newland (1985) surveyed physicians regarding their premedical education. Almost three-quarters favored putting more emphasis on non-science courses. Of the physicians that suggested change, 83% requested more humanities, 42% more business, 10% the addition of computer courses and 7% more exposure to law. The authors conclude that the ability of physicians to recognize the importance and quality of their education often does not occur until after they have completed their medical training and established their practice. It may be up to medical schools to show colleges and universities how to remedy this problem. Simply requiring that certain courses be completed and requiring personal statements cannot ensure that students will be altruistic. It would seem that interviews must carry the burden and so must be taken very seriously.

Considering the role and identity of the physician, the way that we select medical students could not be worse (Ellard, 1974). The practice of medicine in Western societies is seen as a scientific activity, but whether our present scientific course of studies is the best one to prepare physicians to deal with the challenges of medical practice is at least questionable. Students with high science grades usually gain admittance to medical school, but simply having high science scores in a premedical course of studies is, according to Ellard (1974), just about the worst reason for studying medicine. This criterion favors what he calls "convergent thinkers"—those who excel early in their studies, have a primary interest in the physical sciences and are given to technical interests. Such people tend to be generally conventional and to hold authoritarian attitudes. "Divergent thinkers," on the other hand, tend to have artistic and biological interests and to be more unconventional. They have an interest in people and are more emotionally uninhibited. What medical training does is to take in convergent thinkers, train them in science and then expect them to behave like divergent thinkers. This is a recipe for failure (Ellard, 1974).

Students are wary and even cynical about these issues and especially about the rhetoric surrounding premedical education and humanism. A student from the Yale oral history project said:

> Look, you're told from the start that you should never get below a "B." Then they tell you that you should broaden yourself. They tell you to take courses that really interest you. And then they say, "But don't take risks." Risks aren't good for premeds. They tell you in a hundred different ways that to get into medical school you need very good grades. So you can't be a risk-taker. And this starts you

off right from the beginning on a whole life of panic (Viseltear, 1985, p. 38).

A student who had already received a doctorate in literature discussed the problems with the admissions process.

> I think that the selection process here simply doesn't work. We admit students on the basis of how well they did in organic chemistry. Organic?! Getting a good grade in a course like that requires only rote memorization. What will it tell you about how good a physician that person will be? Nothing. We select people for their skill in the basic and physical sciences, but this only guarantees that they'll not embarrass the school by flunking out in the first two years. You see, once we're through the basic sciences a whole different set of qualities are called into play. And these characteristics are as important as the other. It's sheer luck that students possess both. And more often than not, owing to the criteria we've established, we only get the former. We need physicians who are patient, sensitive and wise, but we don't necessarily select students for these characteristics (Viseltear, 1985, p. 38).

Premedical students are getting a double message. Medical school officials say that a broad, humanistic premedical education is essential (as opposed to narrow scientific training), but many faculty members frequently send the opposite message. In 1939 the president of Harvard University said:

> I realize that many deans, professors and members of the medical profession protest that all they desire is a man with a liberal education, not a man with four years loaded with premedical sciences. The trouble is very few people believe this group of distinguished witnesses. Least of all the students (Ludmerer, 1999, pp. 61-62).

Even then, medical school admissions officers knew that the character of prospective physicians was important, but no one knew how to measure this elusive quality (Ludmerer, 1999, p. 62).

Students are told to develop themselves, to expand their horizons and to develop their human side. But to do this is risky for their grade point average insofar as it brings students into new and challenging territory. The admissions process tells them not to take such risks. Thus the challenge is not only to reform attitudes of physicians but to reformulate the philosophy of choosing those who will be admitted to medical school.

Thomas Inui argues that the medical school admissions process provides an opportunity to make medical schools more socially responsible. Good medical school candidates have attributes other than the standard "credentials" required for medical school admission. Individuals who can serve as "citizen-advocates for health" should not have concentrated only on the sciences in their premedical studies. Medical schools needs students who have "innate interest in, and social commitment to, the full array of human institutions that would naturally attract physicians to these kinds of societal-mode roles." The peer interaction that would be fostered by a sufficient number of such students could serve to enhance the medical education of all. Similar arguments could be made for affirmative action programs and programs that recruit to medical schools the children of families who have lived in poverty or rural settings (Inui, 1992, pp. 41-42).

Premedical education offers ample opportunities for development of the humane character and social responsibility required of physicians. Medical schools need to be vigilant in searching for students who have developed this kind of character and identifying them through effective interview techniques.

IV. Teaching Care for the Poor in Medical School

Linn et al. (1987) measured "humanistic attitudes" in postgraduate physicians at two teaching hospitals. This attitude includes such aspects of character as integrity, respect, compassion, empathy and patient-centeredness. The researchers found no relationship between humanistic attitude and physician race, sex, marital status or number of children or history of divorce. In addition, humanism was not related to honor society membership or number of articles published. What was significantly correlated with humanistic attitudes was the number of humanities courses and social science courses taken. Physicians who had worked with the disadvantaged or the elderly or who had been involved in political or social action were more humanistic. The study suggests that humanistic attitudes may already have matured by the time of internship and are not likely to change during postgraduate medical training. This highlights the importance of character formation in medical school and before.

Inui (1992) argues that since medical care is a social good, medical schools have social responsibilities that should be manifest in their missions and activities. He finds the origins of the schools' mission in the notion of a "social contract." If the school is a public institution, the argument for a social contract can be made quite explicit, but even in private institutions a substantial portion of funding comes from public sources and so the notion of a social contract may reasonably be invoked. There are, however, alternative ways of explaining the social contract between medical schools and the communities they serve. One would be a social utilitarian "implicit contract." Health is necessary for all members of society if they are to be productive, and so medical schools have an important utilitarian role in maintaining an essential public good. A third conceptual approach comes from social theorists of the twentieth-century liberal tradition. The basic right of a citizen is to equity—no individual is "more worthy" than any other. Because illness interferes with the affected individual's capacity for participation in the activities of society, medical schools have important roles as "enabling resources" for the citizens of the liberal state (Inui, 1992, pp. 25-27).

Faulkner and McCurdy (2000, p. 347) also argue that medical schools have a duty to teach their students to be socially responsible. A socially responsible individual is "a person who takes part in activities that contribute to the happiness, health, and prosperity of a community and its members." The objective, according to the authors, may vary from place to place, but it ultimately is to produce socially responsible physicians and not just to impart knowledge on social responsibility.

There was a brief period of activism when medical students urged their schools to be more responsive to the needs of the poor who often resided in the shadows of their schools. In the late 1960s, students formed health organizations that provided a national link among students directly involved in serving the poor. But by the mid-1970s this activism had subsided, and the more politically conservative mood that took over has lasted to the present (Ludmerer, 1999, pp. 239-243).

Several national and international bodies have called for medical education to be more oriented toward the needs of the communities that they serve (White & Connelly, 1992). Although it would seem that medical schools have little choice but to serve the needs of the community in which they find themselves, few actually do so. White and Connelly (1992, pp. 4-9) encourage medicine to "reestablish itself as the public's advocate." What this requires is the teaching of "population-based concepts and skills" that will serve the broader needs of the public in contrast to the more traditional individualistic orientation of the physician-patient relationship.

The structure of contemporary health care may serve to undermine such educational efforts, however. Mauksch (1980) argues that three factors affect the social role and mitigate the intended effects of programs that try to improve access to health care for the poor. First, health care continues to focus not on maintaining health but on treating disease. This puts the focus on biology and technology rather than on social and cultural issues. This has changed somewhat since the time that Mauksch wrote, but it still remains a problem. Second, medical care in our society is sought by a consumer rather than being initiated and delivered by a provider. The structures of medical education and the health care delivery system work against the efforts of those who need care but do not know how to gain access to it. Third, the American value system is one that valorizes the idea of individual control over one's own fate. The history of American governmental programs put care for the poor "either in the domain of charity or in that of guilt, but rarely if ever do these programs appear as an expression of a normal, pervasive social responsibility" (Mauksch, 1980, p. 42).

There is controversy about whether medical education itself undermines humanism. Loretta Kopelman (1983) cites several studies showing that medical students become more cynical and less humanitarian during the course of their education. Some students confirm that their education undermines the ideals that motivated them to study medicine. Students perceive the gap between the ideals of the profession and what is actually done. Many students are abused in subtle and overt ways by their teachers and this treatment may be the most important factor in making students lose their altruistic ideals (Kay, 1990). Petrie et al. (1999) found no evidence that students were less altruistic and more money-oriented in the later years of their medical studies than in the beginning. This is good news in one sense, but it is more disturbing when the data are examined more closely. The most frequent wish of medical students was happiness in career and personal life (34%). The second most frequent wish was for money (32%). Altruism came third (31%). Achievement, health, intimacy and self-esteem were the other wishes expressed by 15% or more of the students surveyed. Wishing for happiness in career and personal life is natural and commendable, but as many students wish for money as wish to be altruistic.

Crandall et al. (1993), in a southwestern state university medical school, studied attitudes about caring for the indigent in relation to the number of years of medical training. They found that many first-year medical students believe that access to basic and emergency medical care is a right for all regardless of ability to pay. These students believe that they have a responsibility to care for the poor. By the fourth year of medical school, however, many students believe these things to a significantly lesser degree. They are less willing to provide all services for those who cannot afford to pay and they have a less favorable attitude toward these people. Female students, regardless of year in medical school, are significantly more willing than males to support the provision of care to the needy and feel a greater sense of personal responsibility to provide such care. The authors do not attempt to explain this change in attitude over time and call for more longitudinal studies that would study cohorts of medical students as they go through medical studies. They do rightly conclude, however, that changing the health care system will not necessarily provide better care for the needy. What is needed is a change in physicians' attitudes.

Another group did a study of the type called for by Crandall et al. They surveyed a cohort of second-year medical students in 1996 and again in their fourth year in 1998. This study came up with remarkably different findings. Only a few fourth-year students (8.9%) believed that they would spend half or more of their time working with indigent patients and two-thirds indicated that they would spend no more than a quarter of their time working with indigent patients. When compared with their responses in their second year of studies, 31% more fourth-year students felt "personally responsible for providing care to indigent patients." The factors identified as influencing the desire to work with the poor include a sense of personal responsibility (73.6%), physician role models (64.8%) and previous experiences with indigent patients (63.8%). The authors conclude that attitudes about working with indigent patients are "influenced and solidified" by experience in medical school and by role models (O'Toole et al., 2002).

That change in students' attitudes for the better is confirmed by another study that showed that volunteer service with a homeless population is fostered by education and training. Among residents, participation in a structured program for the care of the homeless was associated with an increase in subsequent volunteer work with the poor. The medical students who volunteered service were more likely to be first-year students, to have previously volunteered in similar settings, to have positive attitudes toward caring for indigent patients and to have fewer discouraging attitudes. The authors conclude that attitudes, perceptions and future plans among medical students are "fluid and pliable and directly influenced by the academic experience" (O'Toole et al., 1999).

If there is a lesson to be learned here, it is that attitudes are shaped not so much by curriculum but through personal experience and interaction with role models. This is how character is formed in medical education, for better or for worse. Medical educators have known this for a long time; they began after the Civil War to reject the passive learning model of lectures in favor of laboratory and clinical experience (Ludmerer, 1999, p. 6). Despite this advantage, medical school faculty have long been distracted from the opportunity to serve as role models. In the 1970s and 1980s, the primary distraction was increasing importance of research (Ludmerer, 1999, p. 309). By the mid-1990s, the deteriorating financial condition of most medical schools forced clinical faculty to see more and more patients. As a result, faculty were less able to spend time mentoring students (Ludmerer, 1999, p. 372).

Attempts are being made to form the proper sort of character in medical school by building experiential learning into the curriculum. One approach uses a workshop focused on discussion of altruism augmented by role playing to emphasize its importance (Gedeit & Murkowski, 2001). Another uses a seminar in the third year of medical school to help students to acknowledge and confront their prejudices. Students attend Alcoholics Anonymous meetings, visit nursing homes, take medical histories from adolescents in a homeless shelter, deliver home care, accompany nurses on hospice visits and provide patient education at a community center for an underserved population. Students discover that experiential learning with proper reflection and discussion helps them to become compassionate toward the poor and other groups toward which they carry some prejudice (Sifri et al., 2001). At the University of California, Berkeley, the "Suitcase Clinic," so-named because it goes wherever the homeless are found, is coordinated on an all-volunteer basis by undergraduate, medical and optometry students. An undergraduate course trains the students and provides the clinic's leadership. A graduate course, open to master's degree and medical students, weaves much of its content into teaching during client conferences in the clinic (Steinbach et al., 2001). The medical school at the University of California, San Francisco, has a two-week elective course for fourth-year medical students in which students work in clinics for the homeless. Students report that the course provides them with role models and teaches them innovative ways to care for indigent patients (Buchanan & Jain, 2001). Such experiential learning is the most effective way to change attitudes.

Carl Taylor (1994, p. 631) argues that international experience can inculcate altruism in students. One objective of such a program is to "partially compensate for the negative impact most medical education has on altruistic attitudes." A second objective is to try to compensate for the "overwhelming materialism of modern medical practice" that the authors see as the greatest threat to idealism. If students are adequately prepared to enter into a foreign culture, are part of a team and receive the proper guidance, they can gain a tremendous amount. Students not only encounter illnesses they would not otherwise see and acquire useful skills, but they develop a heightened awareness of social problems. Physicians who have worked overseas "have their eyes opened" and often notice things in ghetto neighborhoods at home where they have previously driven through in oblivion.

A "hidden curriculum" has always operated in American medical schools. It is concerned with teaching students a proper bedside manner, helping them to see patients not just as exemplars of disease but as human beings and teaching them proper values (Ludmerer, 1999, pp. 70-72). It is this last task—the inculcation of proper values—that I am suggesting is so important as to deserve special attention. The development of a social conscience that actively seeks to help the sick poor is a value that needs to be made explicit.

Accomplishing this should not require the addition of more courses to the medical school curriculum. Thus I am not suggesting a reduction in the amount of science in favor of more humanistic courses. The studies I have cited suggest that the most effective pedagogical methods for achieving what I am advocating could be done within the existing medical curriculum. The key is to get students to see what they are already doing from a different perspective. The greatest challenge may be to find mentors who are willing to use the time they have with students to convey the message that caring for patients is more important than fulfilling economically driven quotas. I have no illusions that this will be easy, but I do believe that it is crucial.

V. Conclusion

We have traditionally wanted our physicians to be both technically competent and humane. To these two qualities we would do well to add a third: physicians must have a social conscience. The idea of the preferential option for the poor is a specification of this social consciousness that is especially apt in an era of increasing commercialization of health care in which the poor can easily be forgotten. If a preferential option for the poor is to take root in medicine, there must be a change of attitude in physicians. This attitude is not easily acquired. It must be developed through the entire educational process—from premedical studies through post-graduate training. Medical education must hold character development to be important. This is a matter that is not easily taught in traditional courses. Experiential learning is apt to be much more effective for such character development. This kind of learning, however, requires the selection of students with the sort of attitudes that are amenable to the educational processes designed to develop a social conscience in physicians. Thus the medical school admission process may need to shift its primary emphasis. Certainly proficiency in the natural sciences is important. But social consciousness that considers the health needs of the most vulnerable members of society is equally important for the good of all our society.

References

Buchanan D & Jain S (2001). Teaching students about health care of the homeless. *Academic Medicine*, 76, 524-525.

Crandall SJS, Volk RJ & Loemker V (1993). Medical students' attitudes toward providing care for the underserved: Are we training socially responsible physicians? *Journal of the American Medical Association*, 269, 2519-2523.

Ellard J (1974). The disease of being a doctor. *Medical Journal of Australia*, 2(9) 318-323.

Faulkner LR & McCurdy L (2000). Teaching medical students social responsibility: The right thing to do. *Academic Medicine*, 75, 346-350.

Gedeit R & Murkowski K (2001). A workshop to teach and evaluate medical students' altruism. *Academic Medicine*, 76, 506.

Ginzberg E & Brann E (1980). How the medical student views his profession and its future. *Inquiry*, 17, 195-203.

Graef I (1977). Decline of altruism in medical care. *New York State Journal of Medicine*, 77, 1454-1456.

Griffin GB (1996). Fallon refused to treat nonmember having heart attack. *Telegram & Gazette*, Worcester, MA. August 2, A1.

Hilfiker D (1989). Are we comfortable with homelessness? *Journal of the American Medical Association*, 262, 1375-1376.

Inui TS (1992). The social contract and the medical school's responsibilities. In KL White & JE Connelly (eds). *The medical school's mission and the populations' health: Medical education in Canada, the United Kingdom, the United States, and Australia*. New York: Springer-Verlag.

Jonsen AR (1983). Watching the doctor. *New England Journal of Medicine*, 308, 1531-1535.

Kay, J (1990). Traumatic deidealization and the future of medicine. *Journal of the American Medical Association*, 263, 572-573.

Kopelman, LM (1983). Cynicism among medical students. *Journal of the American Medical Association*, 50, 2006-2010.

Linn LS, Cope DW & Robbins A (1987). Sociodemographic and premedical school factors related to postgraduate physicians' humanistic performance. *Western Journal of Medicine*, 147, 99-103.

Ludmerer K (1999). *Time to heal: American medical education from the turn of the century to the era of managed care.* New York: Oxford University Press.

Mauksch, HO (1980). Can future physicians be educated to care for underserved people? *Public Health Reports*, 95, 41-43.

Miles SH (1992). What are we teaching about indigent patients? *Journal of the American Medical Association*, 268, 2561-2562.

Nelson AR (1989). Humanism and the Art of medicine: Our commitment to care. *Journal of the American Medical Association*, 262, 1228-1230.

O'Toole TP, Hanusa BH, Gibbon JL & Boyles SH (1999). Experiences and attitudes of residents and students influence voluntary service with homeless populations. *Journal of General Internal Medicine*, 14, 211-216.

O'Toole TP, Gibbon J, Harvey J and Switzer G (2002). Students' attitudes toward indigent patients. *Academic Medicine*, 77, 586.

Ouzts HG and Newland HR (1985). Shakespeare or Krebs? Premedical education. *Annals of Internal Medicine*, 103, 809-810.

Petrie, KJ, White, GR, Cameron, LD & Collins, JP (1999). Photographic memory, money, and liposuction: Survey of medical students' wish lists. *British Medical Journal*, 319, 1593-1595.

Sifri, RD, Glaser, K & Witt, DK (2001). Addressing prejudice in medicine during a third-year family medicine clerkship. *Academic Medicine*, 76, 508.

Steinbach A, Swartzberg J & Carbone V (2001). The Berkeley suitcase clinic: Homeless services by undergraduate and medical student teams. *Academic Medicine*, 76, 524.

Taylor CE (1994). International experience and idealism in medical education. *Academic Medicine*, 69, 631-634.

Viseltear AJ (1985). 333 Cedar Street: An oral history—a chapter in the history of contemporary medicine. *Yale Journal of Biology and Medicine*, 58, 29-49.

Watson DS (1996). In search of the story: Physicians and charity care. *St. Louis University Public Law Review*, 15, 353-369.

White, KL & Connelly, JE (1992). Redefining the mission of the medical school. In: KL White & JE Connelly (Eds). *The medical school's mission and the populations' health: Medical education in Canada, the United Kingdom, the United States, and Australia.* New York: Springer-Verlag, 3-22.

Part III

Examples at Work

8. Rachel Bognet

A Service Mission to Haiti Sponsored by the Medical Alumni Council

> You in others—this are your soul. This is what you are. This is what your consciousness has breathed and lived on and enjoyed throughout your life your soul, your immortality, your life in others. . . . You have always been in others and you will remain in others.
>
> Boris Pasternak
> *Doctor Zhivago*

I. A Project Developed by Scranton's Medical Alumni

For several years, members of the University of Scranton's Medical Alumni Council (MAC) explored options through which they might make meaningful contributions to a region in need of quality health care. After considering several domestic sites, each of which presented challenges in terms of practice venues and insurance coverage, the MAC chose to focus its service efforts in Haiti, the poorest country in the Western Hemisphere. In November 2001, MAC Chairman Richard Bevilacqua DMD, MD, a Scranton alumnus from the class of 1983, sent a letter to fellow medical alumni requesting donations "to initiate a bold endeavor . . . involving hands-on surgical care, primary care and dental care as well as an attempt to begin public health initiatives." Despite a short two-month time frame between the written request and the trip, the response was overwhelming. Very generous alumni contributed $31,480, and most notably, dedicated friend of the University and alumnus, Bernard V. Hyland, MD from 1974, contributed $25,000.

For the past three years, the Medical Alumni Society has sponsored an annual medical mission to L'Hôpital Lumière in Bonne Fin, Haiti. Each year, three physicians, all alumni of the University of Scranton, help to staff the 130 bed hospital, performing dozens of operations and offering many hours in the medical clinics during one week in January. The program also has a remarkable educational component: two or three undergraduate students accompany the physicians, serving as their assistants. These students are thereby offered a unique opportunity to encounter Haitian culture, to learn about medical needs in the third world and to serve some of the poorest people in the world. Those fortunate to be selected are infused with the spirit of service alive in their mentors, an experience that will mark them for a lifetime.

The three participating undergraduate students are significantly involved in planning this service mission. For example, they collect medical supplies donated from local hospitals and medical practices, always in close coordination with the medical ministry that runs the hospital in Haiti. These responsibilities teach the students how to organize a medical service trip, an essential skill for implementing similar missions at their future medical school and subsequent medical practice. Students also educate themselves about diseases such as tuberculosis, malaria, malnutrition, worms and a host of others that run rampant in Haiti yet are only superficially taught in American medical institutions since they are so uncommon in the developed world.

II. The Experience of an Undergraduate Pre-Med Student

The plane ride from the epicenter of the developed world, New York City, to Port-au-Prince lasted less than four hours; yet in that short time, my surroundings changed so drastically that I could hardly believe my eyes. The island of Hispaniola, which Haiti shares with the Dominican Republic, houses a land and culture radically different from my own. I expected to see poverty, but nothing prepared me for the wonder and amazement of the open-air market. In stark contrast to the crumbling buildings and mud-spattered huts all around, in the market stood multitudes of well-dressed people. Not expecting to see them dressed so properly, I could not conceal my amazement, and Dr. Bevilacqua commented, "The Haitians are classy people."

Despite famine, contaminated water, dilapidated shelter, an utter paucity of health care and an illiteracy rate near 85 percent, the Haitian people remain proud and have not let poverty and despair steal their hope. I could not help but recognize the dignity shown by these poor, marginalized and oppressed people. I will never forget the experience of handing food to a wide-eyed, clearly malnourished child and watching him not devour the food immediately but rather run home to share it with his family. From that moment, I immediately felt compelled to join in solidarity with the Haitian people. My encounter with the poorest of the poor taught me that their perseverance and outpouring of love for each other are priceless traits, the kinds of traits I wish I saw more in my own country.

Generosity and care for others are also characteristics of the alumni (Drs. Richard Bevilacqua, Gregory Lynch, Terrence Lonergan and Michael Platt) who so willingly volunteered for the mission, aiding both the poor in Haiti and the pre-medical students whom they guided every step of the way. Through work, conversation and laughter, two other pre-medical students and I became well acquainted with physicians whose Jesuit education had instilled in them the desire to live their lives and practice medicine in a way that promotes service, education and autonomy of others. The physicians were eager to come to the aid of others by using their knowledge to skillfully meet the needs they encountered. At the core of the doctors' service to the Haitian people was an emphasis on education. They spent time working with the Haitian doctors, learning how they might overcome the pervasive lack of resources and technology and also informing them how to perform many lifesaving or life-altering procedures. Our doctors worked in cooperation with the Haitian physicians and students and promoted an atmosphere of discussion and two-way learning on both sides. The alumni physicians also struggled against language and cultural barriers to ensure respect for the autonomy of each patient. The doctors were adamant about informing their Haitian patients of the potential risks and side effects of procedures.

The sound of the Haitian language, Creole, is not the only thing that distinguishes a Haitian operating room from an American one. Temperamental electricity, the reuse of gauze, needles and tracheal tubes sterilized in an anti-bacterial solution and the occasional chicken shooed back through the O.R. suite's entry door help to illuminate the difference between developed and developing world medicine. This contrast became incredibly clear when, on the last day of my first trip to Haiti, I found myself inside a church on top of a mountain, setting up a makeshift clinic in this remote village. As we approached the cinder block church building, I felt overwhelmed by those awaiting care. Those well enough to make the journey packed the pews of the church. As I worked with the local physicians, I learned that horrific road conditions and overcrowded, unsafe public transportation preclude many desperately ill people and emergency victims from the chance at receiving medical care.

The stares of suffering Haitians penetrated me, yet their tired eyes and heartfelt smiles drew me closer. Whether taking their blood pressure, handing them pills, giving them food or simply holding their hand, I received sincere gratitude for any attention I paid to their physical or mental well being. Despite my ineptness while using a blood pressure cuff, the Haitians were willing to give me complete access to their frail arms, leaning toward me as if personal space did not exist and close human contact was the norm. After I took the reading, I wrote down the number on an index card that the patients brought with them. The Haitians firmly held on to their tattered cards and accepted responsibility for bringing them each week to the clinic, thus displaying the value they placed on even the limited amount of care we had to offer. This three-by-five inch card held their entire medical history, which speaks volumes about how little medical attention they receive. Due to the high rate of illiteracy, instructions for taking any prescribed drugs consisted of placing a number in a box below a picture of a rising sun, noonday sun, setting sun or the moon. Yet, even if the patients understand the pictures, in many situations it is unlikely that they will have clean water or adequate food with which to take their medication.

Treating disease in Haiti is complicated by a multitude of factors, including, but not limited to, insufficient education of patients and Haitian physicians, lack of resources and substandard living conditions. As I witnessed health care in Haiti, it became apparent that poverty was inextricably linked to the unnecessary suffering of so many Haitians from preventable and treatable diseases such as tuberculosis, malnutrition, HIV/AIDS and many others. Any person wishing truly to serve the poor must become educated about the underlying political, societal and economic factors that contribute to such widespread disease and complicate prevention and treatment. In his gripping book, *Pathologies of Power: Health, Human Rights, and the New War on the Poor*, Paul Farmer, a medical doctor and anthropologist in Haiti, includes Bertold Brecht's poem "A Worker's Speech to a Doctor" emphasizing the need to work with the oppressed in eradicating the roots of their problems if one is to achieve "pragmatic solidarity" with them.

> When we come to you
> Our rags are torn off us
> And you listen all over our naked body.
> As to the cause of our illness.
> One glance at our rags would
> Tell you more. It is the same cause that wears out
> Our bodies and our clothes.
>
> The pain in our shoulder comes
> You say, from the damp; and this is also the reason
> For the stain on the wall of our flat.
> So tell us:
> Where does the damp come from?

Dictatorships, political unrest, violence and unjust embargoes have wreaked havoc on the public health of Haiti. Immersion trips, which expose students to injustices against the poor, are an integral part of a Jesuit education. It is through interactions with such desperately ill and poverty-stricken people that one most clearly hears the call to serve the health needs of the impoverished and begins to understand where "the damp" comes from.

References

Farmer, P (2003). *Pathologies of power: Health, human rights, and the new war on the poor.* Los Angeles, CA: University of California Press.

Pasternak, B (1958). *Doctor Zhivago.* New York, NY: Pantheon Books.

9. Frank Bernt & Peter Clark, SJ

An Interdisciplinary, International Approach to Justice in Health

I. Justice and the Pre-Med Undergraduate Curriculum

Undergraduates in pre-medical education are challenged by stringent requirements to examine the scientific and medical dimensions of health-related topics. Unfortunately, they often fail to see that these issues have faces and names; that behind the facts and numbers are real people struggling with real diseases and issues. In the spirit of *cura personalis,* we must develop new initiatives to assist students to see the broader issues of faith and justice and how they relate to health care today at the local, national and international levels.

Saint Joseph's University has, over the years, striven to provide pre-medical students with opportunities to explore justice issues. In the past, a large part of the effort was undertaken in the context of the core curriculum and through co-curricular activities. More recently, the effort has become more focused in the interdisciplinary health services major, the focus of which is more directly relevant to the interests of students pursuing careers in medicine and in allied health services. Another new initiative has been the creation of a minor in interdisciplinary health care ethics that allows the students to examine theological, philosophical, scientific, economic, business and interdisciplinary health care issues.

Both programs use service-learning as a means of exploring justice issues in health care. Courses offered through the English Department (literature and medicine), the Theology Department (Christian medical ethics, suffering and death from a biblical, systematic and ethical perspective) and the Interdisciplinary Health Services Department (toward a better death: hospice care; health and society) place students for three hours each week in a variety of service sites that allow them to see theory and practice in a very pragmatic way. They fully examine and critique such issues as economic disparities in health care, racism in health care, issues of informed consent, dying with dignity and quality of life.

II. A New Course: Just Health Care in Developing Nations

Another means of coordinating theory and praxis to show the implications for faith and justice in the health care field involves study tour programs. During the spring 2004 semester, a new course, just health care in developing nations, was team-taught by faculty in the Health Services and Theology Departments. The course focused on issues of justice in health care from the perspectives of public health and medical ethics.

The first several weeks of the semester relied upon Alastair Campbell's *Health as Liberation*, which draws links between the US health care system and American notions of health, freedom and justice. Parallel to reading and discussing Campbell's book, the class explored women's health, AIDS, health promotion, nutrition and disease prevention using *Critical Issues in Global Health* by Koop and colleagues. This book provided a broad survey of issues in public health, introducing students to a wide range of topics from which they might select a problem for their group project.

The first half of the course provided an alternative perspective on what students had heard in previous courses—an effect that the Koop text achieved implicitly. Campbell's book, supplemented by selections from *Questioning the Solution: The Politics of Primary Healthcare* by Werner and colleagues, was more explicit. Both books challenged the students to rethink many of their previously held notions of health care and expanded their perspectives to give them a more global idea of problems facing peoples of the world today. The idea of health care as a human right took center stage, and the disparities that exist between the developed and developing nations not only became more apparent but also challenged the students to broaden their previously narrow view into health care as a basic right for all.

During the second half of the course, students developed the critical skills needed to analyze ethical problems from a Christian medical ethics perspective. Students analyzed cases pertinent to the public health

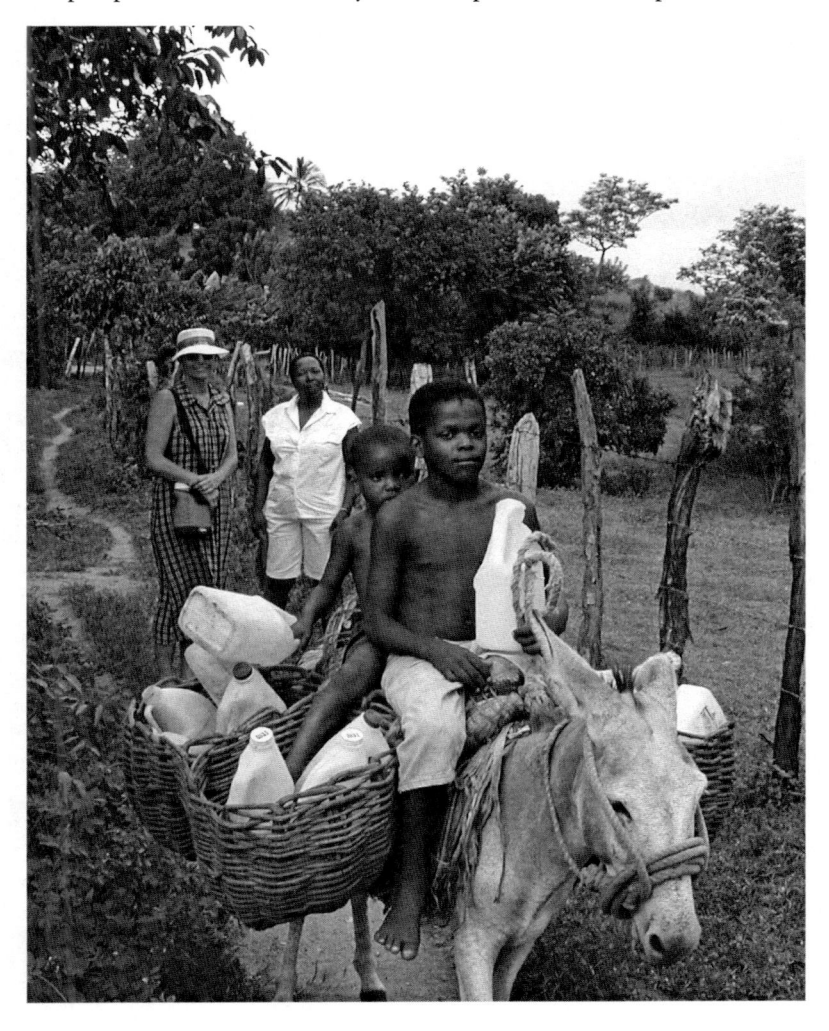

". . . the [Dominican Republic] trip would be better described as a "justice study tour" that *engaged* our hosts rather than simply helping them."
Photographer: Terry Wilwerding

issues they examined in the first half of the course. Cases included disparities in health care, conflict of rights in human experimentation between developed and developing nations, duties of pharmaceutical companies to supply medication to the poor and dying and racism and discrimination in the health care field. They had not only to struggle with their own views of right and wrong but to examine the Christian dimension of each issue. Examining justice, human dignity and human rights from a Christian perspective prompted their rethinking many previously held notions about moral rights and wrongs. Ethical struggles with these issues and challenges from their peers allowed the students to think through them in ways that had been alien to them at the beginning of the course.

Watching this transformation encouraged faculty members to see not only the necessity of such a course in the curriculum but also the need to expand it into other disciplines. The international dimension transformed an initially myopic view of health issues into a global perspective. Dignity, justice and human rights now pertained not only to their neighbors in the United States, but now also to their other neighbors in Latin America, Asia and Africa.

Guest speakers supplemented instructor presentations. The service components of our trip to the Dominican Republic involved evaluation interviews with school children in bateyes near San Pedro de Macoris to assess the effectiveness of a health promotion program aimed at hygiene and hydration. Stephanie French, a Catholic Relief Services (CRS) fellow assigned as liaison for this project, traveled to Philadelphia to describe CRS's work in the Caribbean; the project we would be working on; and the challenges and rewards of forming and maintaining partnerships with governments, businesses and other non-governmental organizations. Saint Joseph's has worked for several years to develop a concrete partnership with CRS in the Dominican Republic. This effort coincided with CRS's recently-begun initiative to work more closely with universities (particularly Jesuit universities) stateside on raising awareness and increasing advocacy-related actions on campuses.

Mark Lyons, a physician's assistant who works in a clinic serving Hispanic patients in North Philadelphia, spoke about his work in health education in both the Dominican Republic and the Delaware Valley.

An Interdisciplinary, International Approach to Justice in Health

His stories and demonstrations illustrated a "liberation pedagogy" approach, modeled on the work of Brazilian educator and liberation theologian, Paulo Freire, and complemented by readings from *Where There Is No Doctor* by Werner and colleagues, that was new and very thought-provoking to our students.

Toward the end of the course, a physician trained in India and a registered nurse who has volunteered extensively in the developing world with Project Smile, talked to the students about health care in their practices. From their own backgrounds, these caregivers helped to prepare the students for their coming experiences in the Dominican Republic. In the ensuing discussion students addressed questions arising from their handicapped reading assignments.

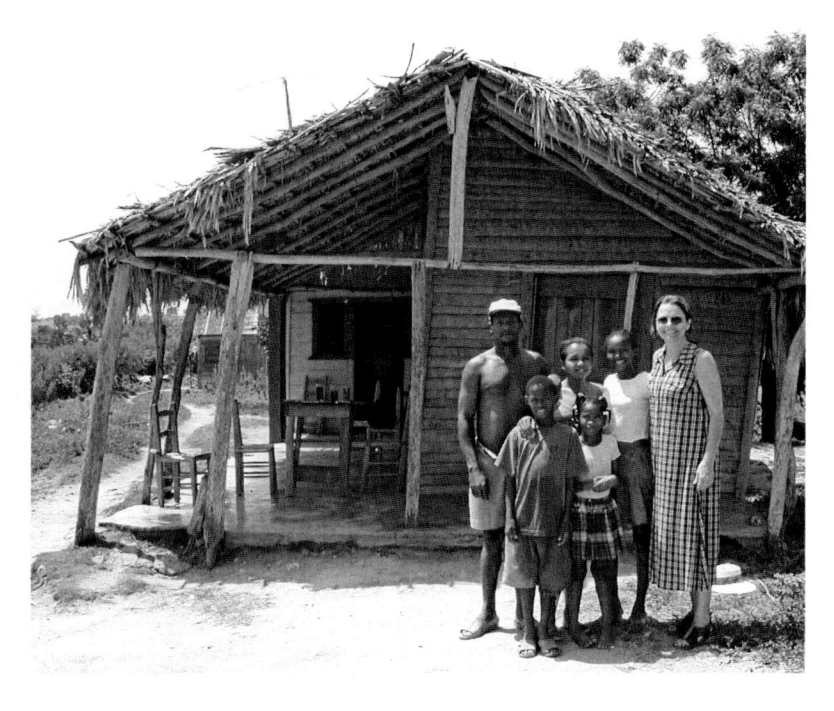

"In the spirit of *cura personalis,* we must develop new initiatives to assist students to see the broader issues of faith and justice and how they relate to health care today at the local, national and international levels."
Photographer: Terry Wilwerding

Although the two weeks spent in the Dominican Republic included service, the trip would be better described as a "justice study tour" that *engaged* our hosts rather than simply helping them. Students sufficiently fluent in Spanish worked with CRS staff conducting interviews and taking photographs at local schools. We spent three days at the Institute of Latin American Concern in Santiago, where students visited children at Hogar Luby, an orphanage for severely disabled children; met with promotoras in a nearby bateye; visited the regional hospital in Santiago; and toured a water sanitation project. In Santo Domingo, we met with staff from Jesuit Refugee Services and Centro Juan B. Montalvo, to learn about the local Jesuit efforts related to violence prevention, AIDS prevention and fighting for human rights for Haitian immigrants. Several of the students traveled to Los Cruces to the southwest of Santo Domingo, to meet with staff at rural clinics about grassroots movements and about the health care challenges unique to rural areas. During evening reflections, students shared with others what they had experienced throughout the day.

III. Food for Thought

The experience of this course has given us much food for thought. First, the ability to capitalize upon partnerships that have been formed over the years contributed to the success of the first iteration of this course. Ongoing relationships with Creighton University, Catholic Relief Services and the Centro Juan B. Montalvo were essential to our being able to further our efforts. Fr. Kolvenbach commented upon the lack of joint cooperation among Jesuit institutions in his Monte Cucco talk (2001). Setting aside such barriers and exploring honest collaboration represents an important step toward "real justice" in pre-medical education.

Second, the balance of service, analysis and reflection is valuable and important. There is a "service impulse" when traveling to other countries that is not harmful in itself but that can easily distract from the many opportunities to learn. In previous visits with groups to the Dominican Republic, we were told again and again that our most appropriate response to the injustices we saw there would be to continue to learn ourselves and to teach others. Suzanne Toton of Villanova University has challenged those involved in service to "carry it further" to include political advocacy. Taking this next step may be especially important among health professionals whose charitable good work is more difficult to transcend because it is so badly needed. That is, Doctors Without Borders and similar groups do wonderful work that needs to be done, but within a very traditional framework of providing health care. Critical to our purpose was the difficult but necessary job of challenging our students to think about how health care might be addressed altogether differently. Expanding their notion of health care on a global level and helping to form their consciences from a moral perspective will create future health care professionals who see acts of justice as more than one-time events. Instead, they will understand that justice must be incorporated into their very being. It is only then that they will be truly men and women for others.

Third, some argue that either summer-long or semester-long programs provide a richer opportunity to transform students. While we would not contest this point, longer programs are not a luxury that students can always afford. The rhythm is certainly different—the two weeks are more intensive both in terms of exposure and reflection. We would argue that in the absence of institutional resources to support summer programs or residencies, briefer study tours are a reasonable and beneficial alternative that provide a valuable international experience and insight into how students can promote just health care for the poor.

This new initiative helps to develop more fully our Jesuit-educated students as human persons committed to faith that seeks to do justice—a justice that extends to all people and a justice that has no barriers or borders.

References

Campbell, A (1995). *Health as liberation: Medicine, theology, and the quest for justice.* Cleveland, Ohio: Pilgrim Press.
Koop, CE, Pearson, CE, & Schwarz, MR (eds.). (2001). *Critical issues in global health.* San Francisco: Jossey-Bass.

Toton, SC (1982). *World hunger. The responsibility of Christian education.* Maryknoll: Orbis Books.

Werner, D, Thuman, C, & Maxwell, J (1992). *Where there is no doctor: A village health care handbook.* Palo Alto: Hesperian Foundation.

Werner, D, Sanders, D, & Weston, J (1997). *Questioning the solution: The politics of primary health care and child survival with an in-depth critique of oral rehydration therapy.* Palo Alto, CA: HealthWrights.

10. Miriam Schulman

Experiencing Ethics: Undergraduate Community-Based Learning in a Local Acute Care Hospital

When Santa Clara University (SCU) students walk into the emergency room at O'Connor Hospital to learn first-hand about the ethical dilemmas of modern medicine, they are actually following a tradition that is almost 500 years old. Like students at Jesuit colleges founded by Ignatius himself, SCU undergraduates are sent out into the community to act on the dictum, "love ought to be put more in deeds than in words" (Ignatius of Loyola).

The O'Connor Pre-Professional Program in Health Care Ethics is a year-long, five unit, upper-division "internship" sponsored by SCU's Markkula Center for Applied Ethics. Established in 1999, the program serves approximately fifteen students a year. It offers undergraduates an opportunity to rotate through various hospital units (Markula Center for Applied Ethics), shadowing health care professionals. They then process what they have observed through biweekly ethical reflection sessions led by Center staff and guest speakers from other institutions including Pathways Hospice and the Jesuit School of Theology at Berkeley.

Students spend five hours a week in clinical observation on a unit. Most often they observe nurses who are involved in daily patient care. Students are introduced to patients and have the opportunity to watch their care over the four week rotations. The students also engage in dialogue with the health care professionals on the ethical issues that arise. In fact the O'Connor staffs have found that the program encourages them to be more conscious of their own processes of ethical decision making.

Often, the first thing students learn is an appreciation for the gift of health. One student reflected: "One of the most important things

I learned is the precious meaning and value of life. Day in and day out, the blessing of being active and healthy is too often taken for granted." Or, as another put it: "It was difficult, yet educational, to enter a department where every patient had a serious history, dim prognosis and yet a very positive attitude and at the end of my shift to exit into an oblivious external world."

Each quarter's reflection sessions focus on an ethical theme such as beneficence or autonomy. Assistant Director of Health Care Ethics, Alice Doyle, who currently facilitates the program, reported:

> Many students became very familiar with issues surrounding autonomy and the right to refuse treatment, e.g., a 94-year-old patient who refused pain medicine because she wanted to be awake and alert. Only with gentle persuasion did she accept a minimum of pain relieving medicine. Another student observed an at-risk patient leave the hospital against advice, respecting the patient's and the family's right to make that decision with informed consent (O'Connor Hospital Board of Directors, 2003).

On units such as oncology, students must confront the limits of medicine. As one found out, "It's hard to come to terms with the fact that medicine cannot stop [all diseases]. That was such a hard thing to realize because for me, the appeal of medicine is the perception that you can 'fix' people. I had to admit to myself that there are some things medicine cannot accomplish."

Another ethical issue, a particular emphasis of Jesuit education, is justice in a health care setting. As one student discovered:

> Patients without health insurance frequently come into the ER. What do you do when you have limited resources? Would it be ethical to just kick those patients out on the street to die because they cannot afford health care? Is it fair to the doctors to make them donate their time? Should the people who do have insurance have to wait longer because of the people who do not have insurance? Clearly, these are sticky ethical and economic issues.

Students gain a new appreciation of the difficult ethical decisions facing the low-income parents who use the O'Connor emergency room for their family's primary health care needs. For example, one student brought to the reflection session the dilemma of a working mother who had been told by the pediatrician that she should keep her sick child at home. The woman took the child to daycare in spite of this advice because she would lose her job if she had to stay home and care for the child.

Because O'Connor serves a diverse population, students have also learned about cultural differences and how they impact medical care. Students are required to read *The Spirit Catches You and You Fall Down*, Anne Fadiman's book on the culture clash between a Hmong family and a California hospital over the care of an epileptic child. As a result Center Director of Biotechnology and Health Care Ethics, Margaret R. McLean, reported, "Many students have remarked on the need to be culturally sensitive and the ethical issues that can arise in cross-cultural medicine" (O'Connor Hospital Board of Directors, 2003).

All of these experiences contribute to the Jesuit goal of training graduates who subsequently make "no significant decision without first thinking of how it would impact the least in society" (Kolvenbach, 1989). They also help students to clarify whether medicine is the vocation for them. McLean noted that many young people are attracted to health care professions because they are interested in science but discover, sometimes only after going through medical school, that they don't really like working with sick people. In the O'Connor program, the students get an early introduction to the real world of the hospital. One candidly reported, "The way I reacted [to watching an IV line being inserted into a patient] makes me wonder if I was really cut out to be in the medical field—a question which I have never really seriously considered before."

Most students are reconfirmed in their career interest, but the program influences their view of the kind of professional they want to become. Being in the ER, one wrote, "makes me realize that when I become a doctor, I need to keep in mind that each individual patient is important and should always be treated with respect, even when they are being difficult." Another student was inspired to think about "potentially directing my efforts too underserved populations as the Pediatric Center for Life does. It is such a rewarding experience and it is a chance to give back to your community as well as to recognize groups of people that society often otherwise overlooks."

Even for those who decide not to go into medicine, the internship provides crucial experience. As McLean said, "Every one of us is probably going to be involved in making end-of-life decisions. In all likelihood, we will manage somebody else's death." The students' confrontation with end-of-life issues at O'Connor helps prepare them for this eventuality. One reflected:

> Death has been on my mind a lot lately. Although it seems unusual for a young woman to be pondering death, I think it has broadened my perspective of life. I have discussed my own wishes for my care with my family, should anything happen to me and have noticed a conscious effort on my part to practice healthy living.

These goals of experiential learning and guided reflection were on McLean's mind when she first envisioned the program. It was, in many ways, the logical outgrowth of her work on an innovative partnership between O'Connor and the Markkula Center for Applied Ethics in the creation of an Applied Ethics Center at the hospital. McLean directs that Center, which provides ethics counsel to patients, families and health care professionals. Over the ten years the O'Connor Ethics Center has been in operation, the relationship has evolved to one in which the Markkula Ethics Center provides ethics expertise and the hospital provides opportunities for community-based learning. Creating the "internship" took several years of groundwork as the program involves putting young people in direct contact with patients. The Center's pre-existing association with the hospital laid the foundation for the program, which requires a trusting relationship with hospital personnel in many different units.

The O'Connor program is one expression of Santa Clara University's understanding of the aim of Jesuit education: to help individuals becomes leaders of competence, conscience and compassion. As SCU defines the goal, "We want our graduates to excel and to bring to their lives an ethical perspective and a commitment to help build a more just and humane world" (Santa Clara University).

References

Ignatius of Loyola, *Spiritual exercises,* 230, trans., Elder Mullan, SJ. http://www.nwjesuits.org/Ignatian/SpEx230_260.html (site accessed 7/22/04).

Kolvenbach, PH (1989). Themes of Jesuit Higher Education. (Key ideas contained in two addresses by the Superior General of the Society of Jesus delivered June 7, 1989, at Georgetown University and Georgetown Prep, summarized and edited by John J. Callahan, SJ.) www.creighton.edu/Heartland3/r-themes.html (site accessed 10/24/02).

Markkula Center for Applied Ethics(2003). *Ethics internship at O'Connor Hospital: A 2002-2003 report.* Internal document.

O'Connor Hospital Board of Directors (2003). *Bioethics report, 2003.* Internal document.

Santa Clara University. Jesuit advantage. www.scu.edu/jesuit/faq.cfm (site accessed 7/22/04).

11. Judith Lee Kissell

Teaching Medical Students about Vulnerable Patients: A Course Example

> "The only ethics issue I can see here is whether prison inmates deserve any medical care at all and if I have any obligation to care for them."
>
> Medical student

I. Introduction

Discouraging as this statement was as we began the fifth iteration of our "Socially Marginalized Patient" class, it points forcefully and cogently to the need for us to teach this course. We are fortunately at a time when the health professions are focusing on access to health care and on how that health care is delivered to the poor and to other socially marginalized groups. It is critically important therefore to give medical students the skills for interacting with a variety of people from places in society that they have likely never been. It is with the necessity for communicating this familiarity with the unfortunate that the Creighton University School of Medicine developed as part of its ethics curriculum the class on Socially Marginalized Patients. This course was developed under the direction of, and first taught by, Dr. Ruth Purtilo, Director of Creighton University's Center for Health Policy and Ethics. It owes much in its conceptualization to her efforts.

The goal of this course is to expose students in their second year of medical school to health professionals and care structures that focus on populations at risk of being excluded from quality health care. Conceptually, the course is organized around the Jesuit (and health professions') moral mandate to give a preferential option to the poor and focuses on what a true sense of professionalism demands as a response to these disparities. The course highlights opportunities for physician career satisfaction in working with such groups, as well as the reinforcement of the ethical and professional obligation so central to maintaining professionalism in medicine today—to care for the poor and/or dispossessed. The basic medical ethical principles of not harming and of honoring justice are more likely to be realized when everyone is treated with deep respect, especially the poor and other socially marginalized persons.

The persons upon whom we concentrate in this class are those whose life situates them so that they cannot participate equitably in the social goods of a society, including quality health care. These persons can be identified by characteristics that include: economic poverty, social status, very young or very old age, mental or physical impairment and challenges and ethnic, racial, religious or gender minority status. In addition, some groups such as immigrants (especially those who have entered or stayed illegally), incarcerated persons and persons with stigmatizing medical conditions (e.g., AIDS), cut across social, cultural and economic strata but may lack quality care if limited to the usual channels of "mainstream" health care.

We teach the class on Socially Marginalized Patients in the second year of medical school as part of the ethics curriculum. These students, otherwise focused on the mysteries of neuroscience, genetics, and other such subjects, have few opportunities for an intensive concentration on such patients. This class provides them the opportunity to focus on the challenges, opportunities and social/ethical issues relevant to working with patients at the social margins of society. Their experiences include a combination of discussions, directed self-study, film viewing, a site visit, interaction with those working effectively in such situations and small group work.

II. The Nuts and Bolts

Although at Creighton University Medical Center this class is taught in the medical school, one of its advantages is its adaptability to other disciplines and to a variety of victims of social discrimination. The class is scheduled in a concentrated week of time that is dedicated almost exclusively to the topic. It would be an ideal setting in which to concentrate on interdisciplinary studies that would include nursing, physical therapy, occupational therapy, dentistry, social work and pharmacy —a future vision that we have for the course.

The Student Planning Committee. We begin with a student planning committee whose main responsibility is to decide the ten to twelve "populations" that we will study for the year. In addition to selecting sites and populations, the planning committee makes suggestions for other activities that occur during the class. Students have suggested breakout sessions with representatives from organizations that serve disadvantaged patients, such as Doctors Without Borders or the Indian Health Service, and they came up with the idea of the Team Report (see below) for sharing their experiences with their classmates. In addition to planning, these students become Student Coordinators for the class. Coordinators are responsible for contacting the course director if there are problems with the site visits; they introduce and act as hosts to the speakers of the various sessions, especially those from off campus; and they help the course director get special information to the other students.

"Populations" that we have used for site visits have included people with physical and mental health rehabilitation needs; mentally retarded children and adults; the homeless; persons who abuse substances; prison inmates; meat packing plant workers (immigrant workers); Native Americans on reservations; poor children; Alzheimer's patients; teenage mothers; adolescents with mental health or behavioral problems; nursing home residents; hospice patients; AIDS patients; and rural residents. The group that will visit population sites is called the "Population Team," or more fondly, the "Pop Team." So, for instance, members of the "Hospice Pop Team," may visit one of three or four hospice sites, either in-house facilities or accompanying a visiting hospice nurse to a patient's home. Students sign up on a first-come-first-served basis for the population they want to visit and study.

The site visit is planned with personnel from the facilities to which the students will go. Many of these facilities are understaffed and must plan carefully for the students' time with them. They approve the days and times and also the number of students they can accommodate. Each Pop Team consists of about 10-15 students, although some groups may be smaller.

III. Structure and Schedule

Introductory Session: The class begins with an introductory session that includes an orientation to the class and the syllabus followed by a lecture or panel. Lectures at this session usually address more general topics related to care for the underserved populations. They may focus on care for the indigent, on social justice issues in general or on cultural issues. Ours have varied over the years, but have included guest speakers, such as David Hilfiker, MD, a physician who has worked with low-income people for 25 years and author of the book, *Urban Injustice: How Ghettos Happen*. We have also used panels of professionals from the community who work with the marginalized and physicians who have served with Doctors Without Borders. Plans for the future include representatives who will speak to students in breakout sessions about serving with the Indian Health Service, Doctors Without Borders, public health service, translation services and the Institute for Latin American Concern (ILAC, a Creighton University organization that sponsors our students at our site in the Dominican Republic for service to the poor in that country; for more information on ILAC, see the contribution by Ayers to this book.).

Literature Study: An especially important part of this class is the time the students give to a literature study to prepare them for the rest of the week. Students are assigned to one of five *topics* related to the population they will visit: Some will study the *demographics* of the population; others the *needs* of the patient/clients; others the *goals* of the facility; still others *policy issues* related to the population; and finally some will research the related *ethics issues* pertaining to a part of, or in some instances the whole, population.

The advantage of assigning topics to a Pop Team is that the combination of the Team's findings contributes toward a comprehensive view of the issues that effect this population. Depending on the nature of the written assignments, students are encouraged to focus narrowly on their topic within the group they are studying. This approach is easier in some cases than in others. For those going to the hospice sites, for example, the topics apply in a relatively straightforward way. But for those who go to the daycare center, prisons or Native American reservations, the possibilities for research topics are myriad. So for the daycare center, students may research malnutrition, language development, AIDS, autism, fetal alcoholism or any of a number of other troubles that may upset these young lives. Nevertheless, the idea of assigning various topics to individuals on the team is an important feature of this course. These students have a reputation, reinforced each year by site personnel who invariably compliment the students' preparedness. They arrive at a site knowing what they want to know and what they need to ask.

Population Planning Session: The Pop Team meets as a group to plan their site visit. The preliminary research conducted by the students leads them to the questions they think to be pertinent at their site visits. Each student brings to the session five questions related to their topic. These sessions are conducted by faculty facilitators, many of whom have experience working with the relevant population. The facilitator of the planning session uses these questions to help the student plan what to look for and what to ask at their sites.

Clinical Issues Session: Physicians who specialize in treating the relevant population meet with the Pop Team to discuss the medical issues that arise for each group. These physicians are encouraged to hold a conversation with the students rather than to plan a formal lecture. We have experimented with scheduling the Clinical Issues Session both before and after the site visit. If it is held before, it prepares the students for things to be alert for during their visit. If after, they are in a better position to ask questions about what they have experienced. Student Coordinators host the clinical participants.

Social Issues Session: This session focuses on the impact of people's lives on their condition as patients. For this purpose, we recruit a variety of participants who are knowledgeable about the population. I purposely refer to them as "participants," since their role is to share and not to lecture to the students. Some examples will explain how the participants are selected. For the immigrant population, we invited a priest who has worked for decades with immigrants from Central America and Mexico; for the school for retarded, we asked a group of parents; for the mental health population, a woman who runs a family support group came; for the AIDS population, patients with AIDS; for the hospice population, hospice workers and volunteers; for the prison group, a woman who runs a program for women former offenders; for the homeless shelter, a substance abuse counselor; for the Alzheimer's population, a family support group that exists at the university.

The possibilities for speakers for these groups are limited only by the imagination. The Student Coordinators play an especially important role for the Social Issues participants, many of whom have little experience in addressing student groups. Since most of these participants are from off campus, the Coordinators are responsible for meeting with them, finding out how to introduce them and for acting as hosts during the meeting. They also take care of special needs. Each year, for example, the Alzheimer's group reminds us that it would be helpful to have a box of tissues handy.

Site Visits: The students visit their particular site for about four hours. This may be in the morning or afternoon. Some sites, such as substance abuse facilities, ask that the students come during the evening when their support groups meet and when residents who are working will be present at the shelter.

Daylong Visits: Two of the populations whom we visit require a different structure. The teams that visit the Native American reservations and the rural health sites spend the entire day. The visits to the reservations are conducted by the Department of Physical Therapy (DPT) that has long experience in bringing their own students to the reservations for clinical rotations. Using the DPT has several advantages for us. First, the department is trusted and respected by the people at the reservation. Second, the DPT faculty members are sensitized to the cultural nuances of the tribes on these reservations and are in a position to inform the students about issues to which they should be attentive. DPT faculty conduct the planning session for this Pop Team before they leave for the reservation. During the course of their visit, the students learn about clinical issues as well as cultural and social issues, so no special Clinical Issues and Social Issues Sessions are held for these groups.

A similar situation exists for the rural health Pop Team. Omaha is fortunate to have two medical schools. Besides Creighton University School of Medicine, the University of Nebraska Medical Center (UNMC) is also located here. Because it is a largely rural state, UNMC has a well-organized program designed to encourage the practice of rural medicine among its own students. UNMC generously sponsors and hosts the Creighton students for the rural health site visit. Although the planning sessions are held on campus by a faculty member with an expertise in rural health issues, once again, our students obtain experience about clinical issues as well as cultural and social matters as they go through the day following the physician or working in the rural clinic. No special Clinical Issues and Social Issues Sessions are held for this Pop Team.

Films: Occasionally, we have made use of films to show to the Pop Teams. We have used, for instance, *Waterdance* for physical rehabilitation; *Girl Interrupted* for mental illness or for juvenile mental health; and *Requiem for a Dream* for substance abuse. The possibilities are endless. Movies both put flesh onto some patient issues that the students may only consider in the abstract and address the affective aspects of providing health care. The disadvantage of using these films is that the students may have seen them.

Debriefing Session: When all the activities have been completed, the faculty facilitators once again meet with their Pop Teams. At this session, the facilitators encourage students to share their impressions and what they have learned from their experiences. This session provides an opportunity for the facilitators to bring closure to the experience as well as for the students to have an opportunity for reflection on all that they have done and seen. On occasion, we have substituted the Debriefing Session with the Pop Team Report (below).

The Pop Team Report: The first Student Planning Committee saw at once the disadvantage of being able to visit only one site. (Our ability to offer more than one site visit is related to the ability of the sites themselves to accommodate the visitors.) The students wanted a way to share their experiences with their classmates. The most efficient way of sharing appeared to be PowerPoint. Each Pop Team is responsible for making a 20 minute presentation. The main instruction is that the presentation cannot be boring! Back-to-back, these presentations make for a long session, but it appears to be a worthwhile wrap up. The activity includes an introductory frame giving the name of each member of the Pop Team, the name of the population and the site(s) the team visited. It is not meant to be an overview; rather the team is to report on aspects about their experiences that most impressed them. Students are instructed to not try to communicate everything but to keep the focus on two or three main points.

IV. Written Assignments

The Scope Note: the "Scope Note" is a format devised by the Georgetown National Reference Center for Bioethics Literature to introduce an inquirer to topic in bioethics that is unfamiliar to the reader. It contains for purposes of our class, (1) a summary of the topic for the specific population the student is studying; (2) an annotated bibliography on the topic about the student's population; and finally (3) a non-annotated bibliography on the same topic and population. Within the class, the purpose of the Scope Note is twofold. First it provides an issues summary and research format that is easy to accommodate within the confines of the Socially Marginalized Patient class, e.g., "What are the issues and what literature is available to study the demographics of the immigrant population?" Second, the information prepares the student to ask the right questions when (s)he visits the site, e.g., "What more do I need to know about the demographics of the immigrant population?"

The Site Visit Report: The second written assignment is the Site Visit Report. This Report is a culmination of all the activities in which the student has engaged during this course. Students can draw on the information, insights and perceptions they have gained from discussions, their literature study, their Pop Team sessions and, most important, the site visit itself.

These written assignments generally provide an analysis and assessment of the effectiveness of the course as well as material by which student participation can be evaluated.

V. Conclusion

Any question about the value of this course is resolved in looking at the students' reflections that appear in their Report. A few examples demonstrate the importance of this kind of class.

> "I found the experience to be interesting and rewarding. . . . I feel privileged to have been able to listen to these patients as they told us their stories. It was reassuring to know that many resources and services exist for AIDS patients."

> "I am very grateful for the opportunity to learn about the HIV/AIDS population. The information I learned from my visit will assist me to become a better physician."

> "I have a hard time expressing what I learned this past week. . . . I learned so much about the pathology of Alzheimer's disease and gained a lot of insight into the disease from our group discussions, especially from the people whose family members have the disease."

> "My experience with hospice was both thought provoking and touching. . . . The nurse emphasized that touching, talking with, and listening to patient is essential. Being honest with the patient is also very important.... This experience has been invaluable to me and has taught me about the part of medicine students do not always learn."

> "This site showed me that services can greatly benefit people with mental illnesses and help these patients through their toughest times. By exposure to such a place I can share what I have learned with others with whom I have interactions throughout my medical career."

The Socially Marginalized Patient course represents our effort to concretize the Jesuit moral mandate to give a preferential option to the poor, to address health disparities and to educate our students about what a true sense of professionalism demands. It embodies the efforts of David Thomasma, who, with Ed Pellegrino, urged us in their *Helping and Healing* to recognize that:

> A healing community must care for those it succors (118) . . . The Christian vocation is quite specifically oriented to a charitable redress of the inequities of nature or circumstance. It is, in fact, precisely to the losers in the natural lottery—the sick, the poor, the outcast—that Christ addressed his personal ministry and his Sermon on the Mount. This is the basis for the preferential option for the poor that inspires the best Christian institutions . . . (121).

Reference

Pellegrino, ED and Thomasma, DC (1997). *Helping and healing: Religious commitment in health care.* Washington DC: Georgetown University Press.

12. Frank Ayers

Creighton's Institute for Latin American Concern: A Unique Opportunity to Provide Dental Care to an Underserved Population

> EDITORIAL NOTE: A version of this chapter is based on a presentation by the author at the Fifth International Congress on Dental Law and Ethics: Rights, Access and Justice in Oral Health Care (July 31-August 3, 2003; Omaha, NE, USA, cosponsored by the International Dental Ethics and Law Society and Creighton University Medical Center). It is reprinted here from the *Journal of the American College of Dentists* (2004) 71(1), 10-12. Permission to reprint was generously granted by the American College.

For almost 30 years Creighton University School of Dentistry has been sending dental students, faculty and alumni to the Dominican Republic through Creighton's Institute for Latin American Concern (ILAC). Representatives from all of Creighton's health science schools participate in this program. The purpose of the ILAC Summer Program is to provide participants with an experience that heightens their sensitivity to world reality and to the individual's responsibility to this reality. This sensitizing is accomplished through an immersion in the life of rural communities in a developing nation. While living with poor families in these communities, participants attempt to enhance the quality of life for as many people as possible through providing basic health care. In the process, we hope to lead participants to a deeper awareness of self and others and to the promotion of a faith-based justice that is both Christian and Ignatian. Participants have included individuals from all major religions and some nonbelieiver. Many dentists who have no formal association with Creighton have participated in the Summer Program.

The Dominican Republic is on the island of Hispaniola in the Carribean, just east of Cuba and west of Puerto Rico. It shares the island with Haiti. Although not as poor as Haiti, it is one of the poorest nations in Latin America. ILAC now has a permanent center and year-round presence in Santiago, the second-largest city in the country. Since the program started, ILAC health care teams have worked in almost 200 villages, mainly in the northern mountain range and along the Haitian border.

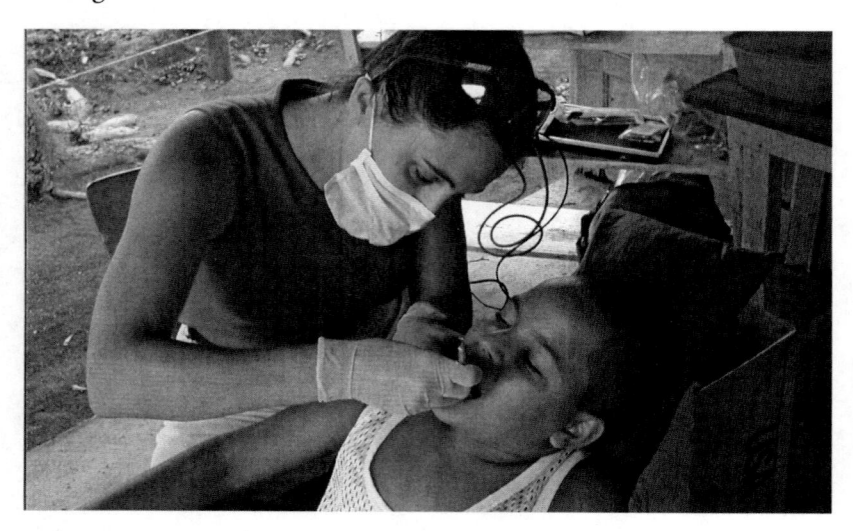

Creighton dental student, ILAC Summer Program
Photographer: Terry Wilwerding

I. The History of the ILAC Program

Father Ernesto Travieso, SJ, a Cuban-born Jesuit priest, is the founder of ILAC and the president of the ILAC Foundation. In 1972 he was working with young men studying for the priesthood at Regis College in Toronto, Canada. In the summer of that year, he began taking Jesuit scholastics to the Dominican Republic. The scholastics lived with families in rural villages, helped the Dominicans with chores and encountered the problems of the poor in a developing nation. The scholastics were encouraged to reflect on their role as members of a global community and view the connection between North American affluence and the poverty found in a developing nation.

In 1976 Travieso was assigned as chaplain for the School of Medicine at Creighton University. He saw this as an opportunity for his modest Summer Program to grow and involve health care students and professionals from Creighton to join the young men studying to be Jesuits in this immersion experience. At the same time the work of health care teams would provide a more meaningful way to repay the Dominicans for the warm hospitality they had been providing the visitors.

Initially, ILAC had no permanent facility in the Dominican Republic. A two-week orientation for student participants was held at a Dominican seminary in Santiago. Participants were originally individuals who showed up every summer, provided some health care and left. At the seminary conditions were crowded and facilities were inadequate. As ILAC grew, leaders saw the need for a permanent facility. In 1985 plans began for the program to build a such a center in Santiago, and in 1991 enough of the building was completed to house the Summer Program for the first time. Since then, ILAC programs have continued to grow: the Center and its staff provide preventive health education programs to designated health promoters from the villages where ILAC has worked; it is the home for Creighton's semester abroad program for undergraduate students; several faculty and staff retreats have been held there; and numerous high schools and other universities have partnered with the program for service projects. Health care professionals from many countries have delivered health care to poor Dominicans in programs not connected to the Summer Program. On January 6, 2004, ILAC dedicated a new 4000 square foot, state-of-the-art outpatient clinic and surgical center. This facility has examining rooms, operating rooms, a pharmacy, dental operatories and a reception area. It will serve poor rural Dominicans who do not have access to area hospitals and professionals.

II. The Current ILAC Summer Program

While both undergraduate and graduate health sciences students participate in the Summer Program, for the health sciences students the program is a credit-bearing selective elective beginning their senior year. Recruitment and application begin in October of the junior year and interviews and selection are completed by the end of November. In addition to a variety of information that would be part of any application, students describe in essay form their understanding of the ILAC Summer Program and their reason for applying and to briefly describe their spirituality. The criteria for selection to the program include the following:

1. Students must be in good academic standing but overall class rank is not a consideration.
2. Students must demonstrate a good understanding of the program and an openness to pursue its goals.
3. Students must demonstrate a willingness to participate in group reflection, group prayer and sharing of self.

A meeting of participants from all the health science schools is held in December. Information about fund raising, inoculations, packing lists, etc., are provided. The cost to students participating in 2004 is $2,400. A special tuition-free Spanish class is held one evening a week during the spring semester for ILAC participants.

During late March or early April, students and professionals attend a weekend retreat held at the Creighton Retreat Center. ILAC staff from the Dominican Republic are on hand and do the majority of the presentations. Students receive a history of the Dominican Republic and a description of the Dominican communities that they will serve and students and professionals are told who will serve each village. Team building and enculturation begin at this retreat. Students leave for the Dominican Republic in mid-June and return around the first week in August.

My particular interest and knowledge comes from the dental school. In a typical year, eight to twelve dental students are selected from approximately 20 applicants. Faculty, alumni and at-large dentists

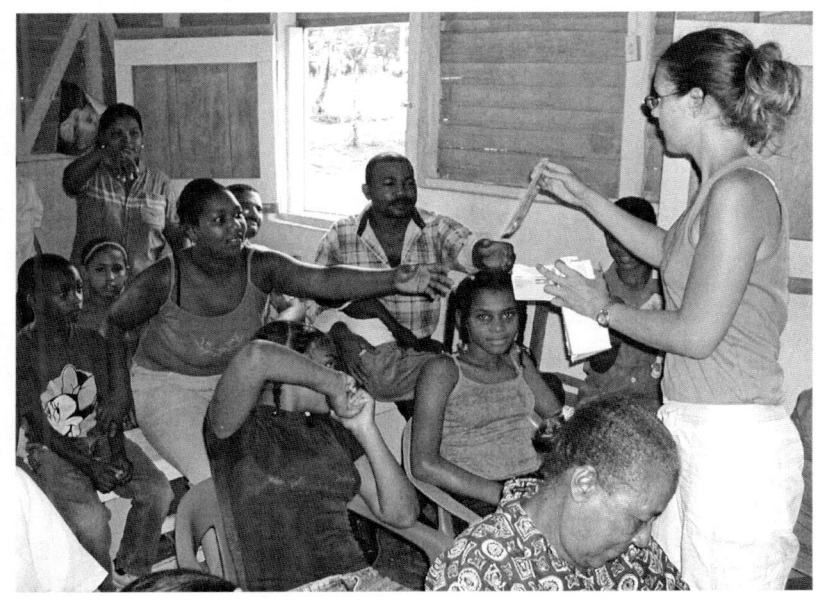

Creighton dental student, ILAC Summer Program
Photographer: Terry Wilwerding

who apply have the option to participate in the program for either a two-week or one month period. It is important for the participating professionals also to have a good understanding of the program and an openness to sharing. Although the main focus of this program is the students, the success of the program depends on the participation of dental professionals. The overwhelming majority of the dentists who have experienced the Summer Program report it as a growth-filled period in their lives.

When students arrive in the Dominican Republic in June, they spend the first two weeks at the ILAC Center in Santiago. They receive classes on the history and culture of the Dominican Republic, Spanish class and motivational talks by the ILAC staff. Teams make a weekend visit to the village where they will be working and spend their first night with their Dominican host family. Throughout these two weeks of orientation, time is set aside for reflection and sharing of what individuals hope to learn from the immersion experience.

Each summer ILAC teams work at six villages. A typical team for each village includes the following:

- group coordinator—usually a student who is an ILAC veteran
- Dominican seminarian—assists the coordinator and provides an important link to the community
- one or two dental students and a dentist
- one or two medical students and a physician
- one pharmacy student and a pharmacist
- one nursing student and a nurse
- two undergraduate students—assist in clinics

The actual immersion into the life of the village is for one month. It is broken into two two-week periods with a weekend break back at the ILAC Center. Different teams of professionals are usually present for each two-week session.

The villages where ILAC teams work are very poor and remote and the people living there have no access to health care, electrical power or indoor plumbing. ILAC brings its own food and water. Participants take meals together as a group to prevent illness, but each member of the group will live with a Dominican family. Clinics are set up at one location in the village and usually operate for half the day. The remainder of the day is spent doing house visits and blending into the life of the community.

The dental clinics are very busy. Time is spent doing preventive education and treating pain and infection. Because of the limits of the community, extractions are the main dental treatment that the team performs. In recent years, gasoline-driven air compressors have been used to power dental field units. The teams also provide restorative services. The dentists supervise students and provide treatment.

Over the years the ILAC health care teams have enhanced the quality of life for as many people as possible in the communities where they worked. Education and treatment are delivered with dignity and personal concern for a segment of the Dominican population that is extremely poor and for whom few others have shown much concern. At the same time ILAC recognizes that it does not possess the resources to affect substantially the quality of the health care system in the Dominican Republic. Providing health care and living with the rural families allows for moments of intense interaction between Dominicans and North Americans that forge friendships and challenge awareness.

The reality of poverty, even one's own personal poverty and limitation, is not lost on most ILAC participants. This awareness has proven to be a life-defining experience for most of the students and professionals who have participated in the Summer Program. A testimony to the power of this experience is the high number of individuals—whether students or professionals—who return several times to the ILAC Summer Program.

There are many programs, both domestic and international, that give dentists the opportunity to provide service to needy populations. The uniqueness of the ILAC Summer Program is that its primary focus is on the individual participant providing the care. They relieve pain; they present preventive education; and they improve the lives of some of the world's poorest. However, in this program, the experience takes place in the structure of a spiritual journey that is calling individuals to look at themselves, their values and their relationship with humankind and the God that (s)he worships.

13. Robin Y. Wood

Bringing Preventive Health Care to a Forgotten Population: A Nursing Research Project about Breast Cancer Screening among Older Black and White Women

I. Mission and Research

Boston College draws inspiration for its academic and societal mission from its distinctive religious tradition. As a Catholic and Jesuit university, Boston College is rooted in a world view that encounters God in all creation and through all human activity, especially in the search for truth in every discipline, in the desire to learn and in the call to live justly together. To this end, the university commits itself to the highest standards of teaching and research and to the pursuit of a just society through the work of its faculty and staff and the achievements of its graduates (Boston College Mission Statement). This distinctive mission moves forward by the university's many services to society. Among these is producing nationally and internationally significant research that advances insight and understanding, thereby both enriching culture and addressing important societal needs. As a faculty member in the Boston College Connell School of Nursing, my program of scholarship is grounded in promoting justice by addressing issues of disparity in health care. My specific interests have been in responding to human suffering by defining where individuals are most vulnerable in the cancer screening and care continuum and by designing interventions that may mitigate suffering by promoting optimal health, comfort and wholeness. Most of my recent research has been directed to breast cancer screening for vulnerable populations of older women, particularly older minority women.

II. Background Information

Breast cancer is one of the most common cancers among women in the United States. The incidence and mortality from this disease increase dramatically with age (Harras, Edwards & Blot, 1996; American Cancer Society, 2001) and mortality is highest in women older than 70 years (Harras, Edwards & Blot, 1996). White women are more likely to suffer from this type of cancer than black women (American Cancer Society, 2001). And yet, mortality rates for African American women have exceeded those of white women in the over 65 age group since 1992 (Parker, Davis & Wingo, 1998; Shinagawa, 2000; Kosary, Ries & Miller, 1995). The most important factor underlying these health disparities is that among elderly women, and specifically among elderly black women, cancer is diagnosed at a later stage (Shinagawa, 2000; Wingo, Ries & Rosenberg, 1998).

Older women are less likely to have mammograms, practice breast self examination (BSE) or have clinical breast exams than are younger women (Vanderford, 1999; Burack, George & Gurney, 2000; Mandelblatt, Gold & O'Malley, 1999; Bernstein, Mutschler & Bernstein, 2000; Breast Screening Consortium, 1990; Rawl, Champion & Menon, 2000) either because they do not know they are at the highest risk for breast cancer or they are not directly instructed by caregivers to have mammograms. Factors impacting screening compliance include patient fears and attitudes about breast cancer in general and screening procedures in particular (Friedman, Neff & Webb, 1998; Phillips, Cohen & Moses, 1999; Lannin, Matthews & Mitchell, 1998) as well as socioeconomic (Madan, Barden & Beech, 2000) and racial variables [Lannin, Matthews & Mitchell, 1998; Lauver, Kane & Bodden, 1999). These problems are complicated by the fact that cancer education and outreach efforts are not always relevant to many poor people who historically are difficult to access and impact with health promotion initiatives (Freeman, Muth & Kerner, 1995).

Although research has not clearly substantiated the value of BSE as a screening strategy (Ku, 2001) key cancer prevention and detection groups continue to recommend the practice as a second line of defense behind annual mammograms and clinical breast exams (American Cancer Society, 2001; American College of Obstetricians and Gynecologists, 2000). However, no benefit derives from practicing BSE unless the self examiner is proficient at the skills for detecting lumps. Teaching these skills successfully requires addressing the special needs of the different populations, including elderly women, in terms of topography of the aging breast and adjusting the procedures to accommodate conditions common in older populations, such as arthritis, visual deficits and loss of tactile sensitivity (Wood, Duffy & Morris, 2002; Wood, 1996). Cancer prevention agencies are therefore urging caregivers to develop cancer educational materials sensitive to age-specific and cultural needs of our most vulnerable citizens (Freeman, Muth & Kerner, 1995; Costanza, Annas & Brown, 1990; NIH, 1993).

III. The Study*

Breast Health Kits for Women Over 60 project was a four year study funded as a Small Business Innovation Research grant (SBIR I & II) by the National Cancer Institute. The purpose of the project was to design and field test age and ethnically sensitive video programs specifically aimed at enhancing breast cancer screening in older black and white women. A unique feature of the kits is that they are designed in separate African American and Caucasian editions thereby targeting the two groups with the highest incidence of breast cancer in the US population with materials appropriate to each group. Based on the conceptual model of Bandura's Social Learning Theory (Bandura, 1977) the intent of the breast health kits was to capture the attention of high-risk women through video modeling of women like themselves depicted in the video.

The video highlights specific age and race risk; benefits of mammography; access and barriers to mammography; issues of mammography discomfort; fear of radiation; fear of finding cancer; step-by-step BSE and the treatability of cancer when it is found early. All actors in the African American video were 60 years of age or older, female and black with voice-over narrative spoken by an African American woman. Actors in the Caucasian video were 60 years of age or older, female and white with voice-over narrative spoken by a Caucasian woman. Although the text is very similar for both videos, the African American edition informs black women of specific risk in relation to similar breast cancer incidence but higher mortality rates than those found in white women. Therefore, the African American video (12 minutes) is slightly longer than the Caucasian edition (10 minutes). These prototypes are the only known videos produced using older women as models for BSE.

Kits were designed to foster interactive practice of BSE skills. BSE skill checks were included as print materials to encourage active drill and practice by the user. The learner scores practice results on a ten-point checklist and tries to improve the score with each use. Other learning and practice reinforcers included in the kits are mini-lump models in black or white skin-tone colors, calendar reminder stickers for annual mammogram and monthly BSE and a poster and educational pamphlet. Narrative explanation instructs the learner in how to use kit materials. The video script was adapted to meet the literacy needs of low education elders.

Field testing was used to test the efficacy of the kits. Two one-hour interviews conducted by trained interviewers in participant homes or community centers provided pre/post-test data related to impact on knowledge about breast cancer risk and BSE proficiency. An eight-month follow-up telephone interview was conducted to determine mammogram compliance. Selection criteria resulted in a volunteer sample of 439 women, ranging in age from 60 to 105 years. Subjects were assigned to intervention (received video kit) or control (pamphlet information only) conditions based on videocassette recorder availability. The majority of participants receiving the intervention were black (77%) as were the controls (78%). The overall sample was low-income and low-education. Almost half (47%) of the intervention group were living below the federal poverty level of $10,000 per annum, but sixty-nine percent (69%) of control group participants were in the lowest income level. Most participants rated their general health as fair or good and most had previously been taught BSE (although 19% of the intervention group and 23% of the control group had never had a mammogram).

IV. The Results

Our results confirm those of other researchers who found that older women are poorly informed that their risk of breast cancer risk increases with age (Bernstein, Mutschler & Bernstein, 2000; Friedman, Neff & Webb, 1998; Madan, Barden & Beech, 2000). Specific item responses revealed that only 25% of the intervention group and 26% of the control group were aware of their increased age-related risk. After using the kit, intervention group knowledge of age-related risk increased to 61% but control group knowledge remained low (33%). Through the use of the video kits participants also gained BSE skills, resulting in significantly higher lump detection scores, rated as subjects demonstrated BSE on a vested breast simulation model. Nevertheless, intervention group participants failed to find many lumps. Seven lumps of various sizes were imbedded in the models, but on average participants missed three to four lumps.

The use of kits did not significantly increase mammography use for these elderly women despite the fact that free and usually convenient mammogram services, such as mobile mammography vans, were in place and available for our participants. Medicare data from the Health Care Financing Administration corroborate that this population historically underutilizes mammography screening (Health Care Financing Administration, 1997). At the time this study was initiated, only 39% of women aged 65 and older in the United States received a biennial Medicare-paid mammogram with lower utilization rates for African American women (31%). It is noteworthy that most of the intervention group sub-sample described in our study was black (77%) and from Georgia (68%) where the recorded rate for receiving a Medicare-paid mammogram within two years was 28% for black women. The fact that 47% of intervention participants in the sub-sample did receive a post-study mammogram represents a substantial increase over state-wide statistics for black Medicare recipients in Georgia at that time.

It is likely that the combination of many factors including low education, poverty, fear of cancer, preoccupation with preexisting medical conditions, some degree of disability or impaired mobility, fear of cancer and declining cognitive status have impacted the low mammography use in this sample. Attention to the pathologies and functional consequences of previously existing medical conditions can distract caregiver attention from the fact that people with disabilities also experience most of the same health conditions as the non disabled (DeJong, 1997). Yet older women, regardless of the extent or complexity of medical conditions, economic pressures and declining cognitive or functional ability sustain the same risk of acquiring breast cancer as age increases.

V. Conclusions

As the amount of time primary caregivers spend with individual patients shrinks, focus on health promotion practices necessarily loses priority to the very real physical needs and health problems of the elderly. Educating older women about their breast cancer risks and the benefits of screening, including teaching them BSE and persuading them to get mammograms, may be impossible goals in the primary care setting when other issues such as hypertension, arthritis, declining vision, diabetes or other medical problems are the focus of primary care visits.

But if the patient is apprised of breast cancer risk and the benefits of screening before seeing the primary care provider, she will be better prepared to ask questions and accept screening recommendations. Trained in BSE technique through video programs viewed at home, patients can demonstrate the skill and receive corrective feedback during the physical examination. Thus the greatest potential for self-instruction video breast health kits may be their use in primary care settings with other strategies, such as provider counseling. Primary care practices, including health maintenance organizations and other managed care plans, can address many barriers to screening by tailoring interventions to patient populations and present them in language and images appropriate for low literacy members or those from minority cultures (Reid, Marshburn & Siddharthan, 1999).

*A full report of this study is published in Wood R (2004). Video breast health kits: testing a cancer education innovation in older high-risk populations. *Journal of Cancer Education,* 19(2) pp. 98-104.

References

American College of Obstetricians and Gynecologists (2002). *Breast self exam.* Education Pamphlet AP145. Washington, DC: ACOG. Retrieved May 24, 2001. http://www.acog.org/breastnibtg/bp145,htm (site accessed 7/22/04).

American Cancer Society (2001). *Breast cancer facts & figures 2001-2002.* ACS Publication No. 8610.01-R. Atlanta, GA: American Cancer Society.

Bandura, A (1977). *Social learning theory.* Englewood Cliffs, NJ: Prentice-Hall.

Bernstein, J, Mutschler, P & Bernstein, E (2000). Keeping mammography referral appointments: Motivation, health beliefs, and access barriers experienced by older minority women. *Journal of Midwifery & Women's Health,* 45, 308-313.

Boston College. Mission Statement. http:/www.bc.edu/offices/mission (site accessed 7/22/04).

Breast Screening Consortium (1990). Screening mammography-a missed opportunity? Results of the NCI Breast Cancer Screening Consortium and National Health Interview Survey Series. *Journal of the American Medical Association,* 264, 54-58.

Burack, RC, George, J & Gurney, JG (2000). Mammography use among women as a function of age and patient involvement in decision-making. *JAGS,* 48, 817-821.

Costanza, M, Annas, G, Brown, M, et al. (1990). Supporting statements and rationale: Forum for breast cancer screening in older women. *J Gerontol.,* 47(Special issue) 7-15.

DeJong, G (1997). Primary care for persons with disabilities. *Am J Phy Med & Rehab.,*76(Suppl) s2-s8.

Freeman, H, Muth, B & Kerner, J (1995). Expanding access to cancer screening and clinical follow-up among the medically underserved. *Cancer Practice,* 3, 19-30.

Friedman, L, Neff, N, Webb, J et al. (1998). Age-related differences in mammography use and in breast cancer knowledge, attitudes, and behaviors. *J Cancer Educ.,* 13, 26-30.

Harras, A, Edwards, BK, Blotm, WJ, et al. (eds). (1996). *Cancer rates and risks*. NIH Publication 96-691. 4th ed. Bethesda, MD: National Cancer Institute.

Health Care Financing Administration (1997). *Mammography screening rates 1994-95.* Washington, DC: HCFA

Kosary, C, Ries L & Miller, B (1995). *SEER cancer statistics review, 1973-1992.* NIH Publication # 95-2789. Bethesda, MD: National Cancer Institute.

Ku, Y (2001). The value of breast self-examination: Meta-analysis of the research literature. *Onc Nurs For,* 28, 815-822.

Lannin, DR, Matthews, HF, Mitchell, J et al. (1998). Influence of socioeconomic and cultural factors on racial differences in late-stage presentation of breast cancer. *Journal of the American Medical Association,* 279, 1801-1807.

Lauver, D, Kane, J, Bodden, J et al. (1999). Engagement in breast cancer screening behaviors. *Onc Nurs For.,* 26, 545-554.

Madan, AK, Barden, CB, Beech, B, et al. (2000). Socioeconomic factors, not ethnicity, predict breast self-examination. *The Breast Journal,* 6, 263-266.

Mandelblatt, JS, Gold, K & O'Malley, AS (1999). Breast and cervical cancer screening among multiethnic women: Role of age, health, and source of care. *Prev Med.,* 28, 418-425.

NIH (1993). *Proceedings: Secretary's Conference to Establish a National Action Plan on Breast Cancer.* Bethesda, MD: National Institutes of Health.

Parker, SL, Davis, KJ, Wingo, PA, et al. (1998). Cancer statistics by race and ethnicity. *CA Cancer J Clin.,* 48, 31-48.

Phillips, J, Cohen, M & Moses, G (1999). Breast cancer screening and African American women: Fear, fatalism, and silence. *Onc Nurs For.,* 26, 561-571.

Rawl, SM, Champion, VL, Menon, U et al. (2000). The impact of age and race on mammography practices. *Health Care for Women International,* 21, 583-587.

Reid, WM, Marshburn, J & Siddharthan, K. (1999). Managed care organizations and mammography: Opportunities to serve underserved women. *Women & Health,* 28, 13-28.

Shinagawa, SM (2000). The excess burden of breast carcinoma in minority and medically underserved communities. *CA Supplement.,* 88, 1217-1223.

Vanderford, V (1999). Older women and mammography: Factors influencing their attitude. *Ger Nurs.,* 20, 257-259.

Wingo, PA, Ries, LAG, Rosenberg, HM et al. (1998). Cancer incidence and mortality, 1973-1995. *Cancer*, 82, 1197-1207.

Wood, R, Duffy, M, Morris, S et al. (2002). The effect of an educational intervention on promoting breast self-examination in older African American and Caucasian women. *Onc Nurs For.*, 29, 1081-1090.

Wood, R (1996). Breast self-examination proficiency in older women: Measuring the efficacy of video self-instruction kits. *Ca Nurs.*, 19, 429-436.

14. Rosanna DeMarco & Anne Norris

Women's Voices Women's Lives: A Web-Based HIV Prevention Film Project

I. The Background

In 2001 a collaborative relationship evolved among Boston College's William F. Connell School of Nursing colleagues, Rosanna DeMarco, Anne Norris and videographer, C. Abraham Minnich. Their partnership, integrating clinical, research and technological expertise led to an innovative HIV prevention film project and interactive website directed toward inner-city African American teen girls and women and the providers who care for them. The project is an exemplar of a community-based, consumer driven undertaking that succeeded because of the commitment of all parties to make health prevention meaningful and relevant to the poor and underserved.

The research and activity backgrounds of DeMarco and Norris were of special significance to the design and success of the project. Both had extensive experience working with community groups that had relevance for HIV prevention. Both had conducted research that is culturally relevant and gender sensitive—much of it with women of color. Norris has studied the sexual behavior of adolescents and young adults for more than fifteen years. Her research includes studies with low-income African American, Latino and Anglo youth. She has extensive background in the study of risky sex behavior, and she is particularly interested in how culture and gender influence this behavior. Her recent work with low income youth has resulted in development of abstinence self-efficacy and behavior measures and also provided questions and issues for the threaded discussion feature of the web-based HIV prevention intervention project. She is the clinical supervisor for a Ryan White-funded counseling program for HIV-seropositive Haitian Americans and immigrants.

Over the past seven years DeMarco has focused on African American women who are HIV-seropositive. She is a cofounder of a community-based collaboration with women living with HIV in the inner city of Boston and HIV service organizations called the "Healing Our Community Collaborative" (HOCC). This group created projects

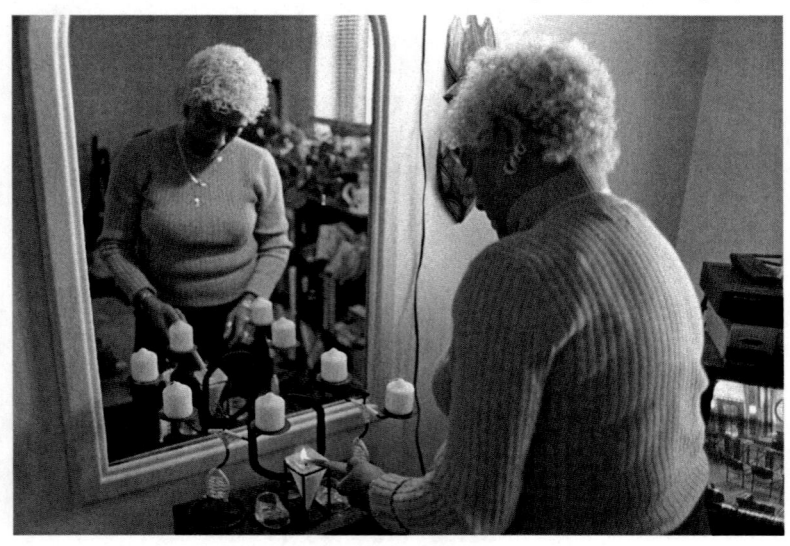

"I would like to think that in a perfect world, I would have liked me without picking up a drug or a drink, and having used a condom." Catherine.
Photographer: Chad Minnich

planned, presented and evaluated by inner-city women living with HIV/AIDS as well as by representatives from HIV service organizations and medical care centers. DeMarco worked with the Silencing the Self Scale, an instrument that measures the degree to which women silence their voices in important relationships. The focus on "silence" explores the dis-empowerment of women and provides concrete tools for both healing and empowerment. The project encouraged African American women to talk more about how they learned to neglect their own care through silence. The women described actions that resulted in poor self-esteem and negative feelings about their lives including the stigma of being poor, living in the inner city and dealing with being HIV-seropositive. These same women expressed a desire to reach out to teen girls in their community so that these young women could avoid the pain and suffering of living with HIV.

In January 2002, DeMarco, Norris and Minnich began filming the stories of four African American women's experiences of living with HIV. The film project was a unique collaboration between these women, the academics and the artist. Most important, it was initiated by these women. They approached DeMarco to help them make an HIV prevention film that would speak to the young women in their community. The stories told about the negative effect of HIV on the women's lives and offered advice to adolescents in their community about risky, versus safer, sex behavior. Thus arose the notion of an inter generational intervention for an African American community threatened by rising rates of HIV infection, specifically among teen girls.

The various themes that emerged in the filming were a product of the women's own personal experiences, as well as their responses to remarks and questions posed by DeMarco and Norris based on their previous research. Themes included finding out that one is HIV-seropositive; emotions and stigma associated with being HIV-seropositive; coping with the many complications of HIV, such as medications, side effects and monitoring oneself or one's children; how women silence and thus dis-empower themselves; and how life does go on so that those with HIV can have a satisfying life despite their condition.

II. The Web-Based Intervention Project

DeMarco wanted to make the film accessible to youth and so the team began working to provide this access in a way that would be safe and effective. With the help of Boston College, which provided a research incentive grant and a research fellowship for one semester, the team developed a web-based HIV prevention program that uses a secure WebCT internet site. The WebCT program was designed to include activities that reinforce and build upon the messages inherent in the film. The film itself was digitalized into five five-minute clips that could be easily viewed over the internet.

The first component of the web-based intervention contains clips from the film and a series of topical links so that adolescents working with the intervention site, can "read more about it" if they want to at their leisure. They can also click on unfamiliar terms for more information. For example, one of the women in the film uses the term "lipodystrophy" when she talks about side effects of HIV medications.

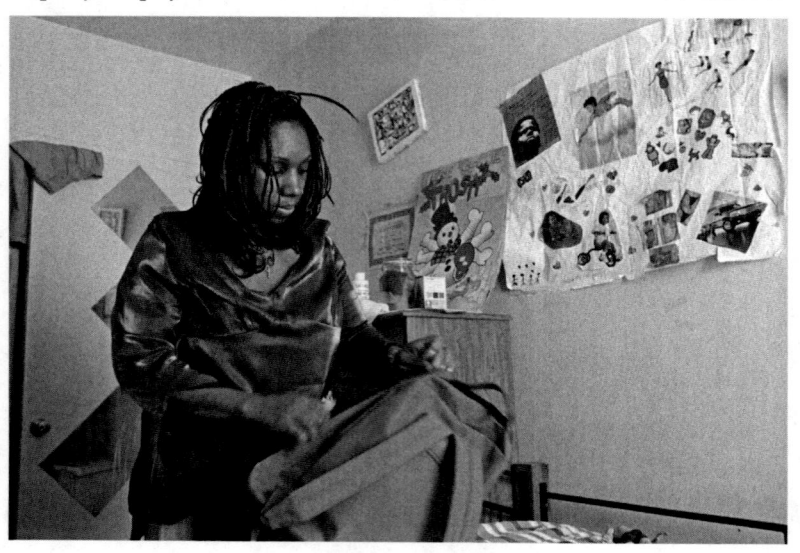

"I felt that I was one of those dent cans on the shelf—that I was damaged ... nobody was ever gonna love me." Tona
Photographer: Chad Minnich

Viewers can find out that "lipodystrophy" means a fat redistribution, resulting from protease inhibitor medications used in HIV treatment that the women consider unsightly.

The second component is interactional. It involves a threaded discussion that allows participants to ask questions of the women speakers and allows the women speakers and the academics to pose to the participants issues and situations related to safe sex behaviors, intentions and attitudes. The intent is to help teen girls develop tangible ways for dealing with peer pressure and norms and for enhancing their own understanding of HIV/AIDS in relation to prevention behaviors.

HIV/sex educators from the Boston Public Schools and alternative education and residency sites met with the DeMarco and Norris to explore use of the web-based program. Each made a commitment to the project and acknowledges the need for having HIV-seropositive women from their communities assist with HIV education. They agree that the program provides advantages over traditional classroom approaches because it affords private, self-directed and self-paced learning for the adolescent while using an interesting and accessible medium. Most important, the web-based approach allows adolescents to review material and return to it as they feel a need to clarify or further their learning of HIV prevention skills.

We are currently seeking funding to support pilot testing comparing the use of the WebCT site between two high schools situated in the same community. With the advice of professional focus groups and grant funding from the Massachusetts Department of Health AIDS

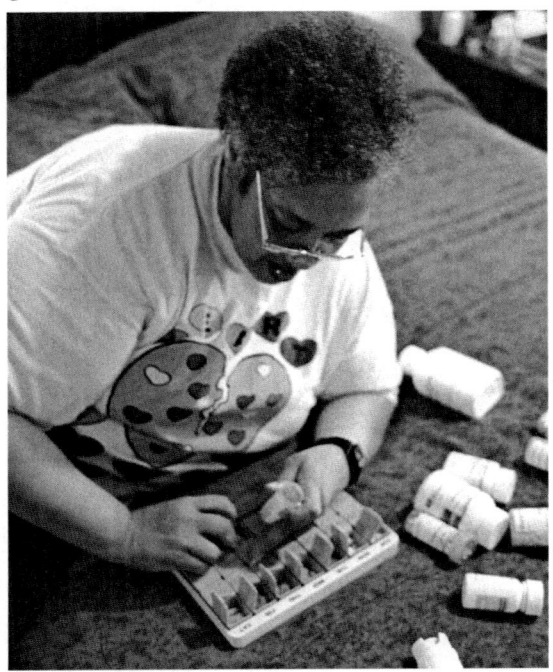

"What brought me to be HIV positive? I am a victim of silencing the self. I grew up believing that I was supposed to do what people said." Sandra
Photographer: Chad Minnich

Bureau, we have edited the teen version of the film and now have women's and provider's versions that include curricula for women at risk, women living with HIV and those that offer them health care. Those interested in viewing a clip of the film portion of the intervention can do so at http://webct.bc.edu:8900. The ID and password are "guest48" (no spaces).

References

DeMarco, R, Bright, H & Johnsen, C (2004). Healing our community collaborative—HOCC: A nurse-led peer-driven service project for women living with HIV. *Massachusetts Report on Nursing, The Official Publication of the Massachusetts Association of Registered Nurses Inc,* 2(1) 12.

Johnson, C (2003). Taking action in communities: Women living with HIV lead the way. *Journal of Community Health Nursing,* 20(1) 51-62.

Johnson, C, Fukuda, D & Deffenbaugh, O (2001). Content validity of a scale to measure silencing and affectivity among women living with HIV/AIDs. *Journal of Association of Nurses in AIDS Care,* 12(4) 49-60.

Lynch, MM & Board, R (2002). Mothers who silence themselves: Clinical implications for women living with HIV/AIDS and their children. *Journal of Pediatric Nursing,* 17(2) 89-95.

Miller, K, Patsdaughter, C, Grindel, C & Chisholm, M (1998). From silencing the self to action: Experiences of women living with HIV/AIDS. *Women's Health Care International,* 19(6) 539-552.

Ford, K & Norris, AE (1996). Sexually transmitted diseases: Experiences and risk factors among urban, low income, African American Hispanic youth. *Ethnic Health,* 1(2) 175-184.

Jack, DC (1991). *Silencing the self.* Cambridge, MA: Harvard University Press.

Norris, AE (1988). Cognitive analysis of contraceptive behavior. *Image,* 20, 135-140. In NJ Kelley, MD Brot, KE Moe & K Dahl (eds.) (1992). *The complexities of women: Integrative essays in psychology and biology.* Dubuque, IA: Kendall/Hunt Publishing.

———, & Beaton, MM (2002). Condom knowledge of adolescents at risk for HIV, nursing students and education students: Who knows more? *The American Journal of Maternal Child Health Nursing,* 27, 103-108.

———, Clark, LF & Magnus, S (2003). Sexual abstinence and the Sexual Abstinence Behavior Scale. *Journal of Pediatric Health Care,* 17, 140-144.

———, & Devine, PG (1992). Linking pregnancy concerns to pregnancy risk avoidant action: The role of construct accessibility. *Personality and Social Psychology Bulletin,* 18, 118-127.

———, & Ford, K (1994). Associations between condom experiences and beliefs, intentions, and use in a sample of urban, low income, African American and Hispanic youth. *AIDS Education and Prevention,* 6, 27-39.

———, & Lopez DeVictoria, D (1998). Measuring the ability to postpone sex: Abstinence self-efficacy. Paper presented at the annual meeting of the American Psychological Association, San Francisco, CA.

Phillips, RE & Norris, AE (2003). A survey of sexual risk behavior & condom use in males in U.S. Navy. *Navy Medicine,* 94, 26-29.

Ruiz, MS, Gable, AR, Kaplan, EH, Stoto, MA, Fineberg, HV & Trussell, J (2001). No time to lose: Getting more from HIV prevention. Washington, DC: The National Academies Press.

Williams, SS, Norris, AE & Bedor, MM (2003). Sexual relationships, condom use, and concerns about pregnancy, HIV/AIDS, and other sexually transmitted diseases. *Clinical Nurse Specialist,* 17, 89-94.

15. Marylou Yam

Survivors of Intimate Partner Abuse: A Nursing Research Project

I. Justice and Nursing Research

Kolvenbach (2000) has asserted that a basic tenet of Jesuit education is the promotion of social justice. The American Association of Colleges of Nursing (1998) also recognizes justice as an essential element of professional nursing education. According to the AACN (1998), social justice for nurses means working to assure equality of treatment and access to health care. In order to prepare nurses who are equipped to be effective advocates for social betterment, content and learning experiences aimed at caring for the poor, the uninsured and the marginalized must be a necessary component of nursing curricula at Jesuit institutions. Faculty in Jesuit nursing schools must emphasize social justice in their research endeavors and should examine their research in light of the Jesuit university's mission of social responsibility. Nursing research can lead to the evaluation of interventions and the initiation of changes in practice and policy. Thus, nursing research can be a means to effecting social change and to addressing the concerns, needs and interests of the oppressed.

Undergraduate and graduate nursing students should be involved in research activities and projects that are connected to social betterment. Such learning experiences will raise students' awareness regarding their social responsibility and enable them to acquire the knowledge and skill required to apply their research to the concern of social justice. In this chapter I describe a research project on survivors of intimate partner abuse. It shows that research can incorporate seemingly exclusive objectives: (1) I have a very strong personal commitment to this project; (2) it is also part and parcel of the Society's social justice mission; (3) it matches my specific knowledge and skills as a nurse-researcher; (4) it enables a scientific assessment of the effectiveness of a therapeutic intervention designed for this population; (5) and it will even yield immediate practical outcomes in the area of health promotion education for battered women.

II. The Proposed Study: An Intervention to Increase Self-Efficacy and Health Promotion Behaviors and Decrease Depression among Women Who Have Experienced Intimate Partner Abuse*

A national study estimates that at least four million women are physically abused each year in the United States (Plichta, 1996). Battered women have been identified as a "vulnerable population" (Tyson & Fleming, 1999), that is, a group that has increased risk and susceptibility to adverse health outcomes (Flaskerud, 1998). An abundance of literature documents the physical and psychological problems experienced by women living in a violent relationship (Campbell, 2002). Women who have been abused have a 50% to 70% increase in gynecological, central nervous system and stress-related problems (Campbell et al., 2002). In addition, these women display increased symptoms and illnesses related to chronic stress, such as gastrointestinal disorders (Campbell et al, 2002) and cardiovascular problems (Coker, Smith, Bethea, King & McKeown, 2000).

In the category of psychological sequelae, depression is one of the most common disorders that survivors of abuse experience (Campbell, 2002). Research also shows that abused women are more stressed and have less ability to care for themselves than non-battered women (Campbell & Soeken, 1999). Moreover, abused women are at risk for under-treatment. Although abused women are significantly more likely to report their health as fair or poor and more likely than non-abused women to say they need medical care, they do not seek it (Campbell & Soeken, 1999).

As Welie explains elsewhere in this volume, the promotion of justice demands analyzing the reasons for inequities in health care and addressing them. So we see that for many battered women, economic hardship makes health care inaccessible and unaffordable. Fear, embarrassment (Rodriguez, Quiroga, Skupinki & Bauer, 1996), ineffective communication and negative experiences with health care professionals (Rodriguiz et al., 1996; Yam, 2000) may also contribute to the under-use of health services.

Several factors, including personal strengths and inner resources such as self-efficacy (Dutton, 1992) can mediate and ameliorate the impact of abuse as well as the woman's ability to protect herself and her children. Self-efficacy is the belief that one can perform the specific behavior necessary to achieve goals. It determines whether one will engage in that behavior (Bandura, 1977) and it enables self-management. Furthermore, self-efficacy has been linked to a decrease in depression (Bandura, 1982) and to the promotion of health behavioral change (Baggett, 2001; Maibach & Murphy, 1995).

Abused women face a myriad of issues in addition to the abuse itself, such as personal safety, self-healing and living arrangements. As they deal with these challenges, they need to maintain their psychological well-being and their physical health. While I could find no study that examined the effects of an intervention on self-efficacy, depression or health promotion behaviors among abused women, related concepts such as self-esteem (Campbell & Soeken, 1999) and self-care agency (Lempert, 1996) indicate the need to examine interventions that can increase the personal strengths of abused women.

The proposed investigation aims at testing an enhancement intervention in order to examine its effect on self-efficacy, perceived ability to implement health promotion behavior and to reduce depression among battered women. I will use Bandura's self-efficacy theory to guide this study. Bandura (1997) explains that self-efficacy influences health behaviors because people must believe they can master and maintain health promoting activities in order to exert the effort required to be successful. Moreover, Bandura (1995) asserts that self-efficacy influences affective states. An individual's belief in his/her ability to cope affects how much stress and depression (s)he experiences—in other words, low self-efficacy can lead to depression. Owing to the violence in their lives, abused women must cope with the stress of living in a violent relationship. Thus, efforts to enhance the battered woman's self-efficacy may moderate the effects of stress and depression and enable her to cope more effectively.

This theory provides a rationale for a supportive education intervention that enables development of self-efficacy and provides an incentive for behavioral change. According to Bandura (1977, 1997), enhancement of this ability is based on four sources of information: performance accomplishments (practicing), vicarious learning (role modeling/learning from others), verbal persuasion and self appraisal of emotional and physiological responses. Each component will be incorporate into the intervention.

The study uses a quasi experimental, pre-/post-test design and non-probability convenience sampling. The experimental group will receive the self-efficacy enhancing intervention in addition to the existing services that the shelter or their community out-reach programs provide. The control group will receive only the existing services provided by the site.

For this purposes of this study, a "battered woman" is defined as a woman in an intimate, cohabiting, heterosexual relationship who has been subjected to physical abuse on more than one occasion by a male partner. Additional criteria for participation will be the ability to speak and read English, completion of at least an elementary education and willingness to complete the intervention sessions. Since pregnant women have different needs related to sleep, nutrition and health promotion, they will not be permitted to participate. Participants will volunteer for the study and sign a consent form prior to their involvement. Approval for this study has been obtained from the Saint Peter's College Institutional Review Board.

Kolvenbach (2000) has urged Jesuit faculty to collaborate with persons in church and social settings who focus on seeking justice. Thus we have sought three battered women's shelters to participate in this investigation. Input was sought in the planning and design of the study from shelter staff as well as from the consultants, one of whom is an internationally known advocate for battered women. We will also solicit feedback from these individuals during the intervention.

The intervention consists of six–two hour group sessions. Each session has a planned agenda with specified objectives, content and activities. Overall the intervention seeks to strengthen the women's self-efficacy by increasing their ability to problem-solve and to promote their own safety, health-related and stress management activities. In order to facilitate efficacy enhancement strategies, the intervention will be carried out in groups. Group size will range from a minimum of five persons to a maximum of ten—a structure intended to break the feeling of isolation for these women. They will be able to observe each other, role play, validate experiences and give and receive information and support within their groups.

Elsewhere in this volume, Welie points out that the poor and vulnerable are often "objects of medical teaching and research." But in this study the women will be seen rather as participants, strong individuals and survivors. The group intervention is intended to empower the women, mobilize their self-determination and validate their experiences. Wood and Middleman (1992) explain that empowerment "involves helping people to develop skills, knowledge and influence that makes it possible for them to gain access to money and resources" (p. 83). These women will, for example, practice assertive communication techniques as well as discuss ways in which they can effectively navigate the health care system in order to access needed resources. They will have a chance to help themselves and help each other. They will have a safe place to learn and to express their voices.

The group sessions will be led by the principal investigator or one of two doctorally prepared nurses familiar with the needs of abused women and Bandura's theory and principles. The principal investigator, as well as the two nurses, have worked with battered women in their clinical practices.

Self-efficacy will be measured by the 30-item Self-efficacy Scale (Sherer, et al., 1982). This instrument consists of two sub-scales, general and social self-efficacy. General self-efficacy measures the feeling that individuals have about their ability to perform tasks based on prior experiences. Social self-efficacy assesses the belief a person possesses about her or his ability to establish interpersonal relationships. Perceived ability to implement health promoting behavior will be measured with the 28-item Abilities for Health Practices Scale (Becker, Stuifbergen, Oh & Hall, 1993). The tool assesses health-promoting abilities in four areas: nutrition, exercise, psychological well-being—stress management and interpersonal relationships and health responsibility—getting health-related assistance and information (Becker et al., 1993). Depression will be measured using the 21-item Beck Depression Inventory (Beck, 1972). The Beck Depression Inventory measures the presence and degree of depression in adolescents and adults.

At the conclusion of the intervention, a questionnaire including both open- and close-ended questions will give the women a chance to evaluate the helpfulness of the intervention. Thus, the women will participate in helping to shape the intervention for future use. Their feedback will possibly create a new intervention that reflects their concerns, and it will provide insight into the usefulness of the self-efficacy enhancement techniques.

Demographic data and test scores will be entered into a computerized Statistical Package for the Social Sciences (SPSS) version 11.0. The t-test statistic ($p<.05$) will be used to compare the pre and post test scores of the women in the study groups on the Self-Efficacy Scale, Self-Perceived Abilities to Perform Health Promotion Behaviors Scale and the Beck Depression Inventory. We will test the research hypotheses ($p<.05$) using the Analysis of Variance (ANOVA) and employ content analysis to analyze the qualitative data. The findings of this study may show that an intervention aimed at increasing personal strengths may enable abused women to make healthy choices, alleviate depression and possibly reduce their vulnerability to potential physical and psychological consequences of violence.

* This proposal was selected to receive the Rosemary Berkel Crisp 2003 Research Award from Sigma Theta Tau International. The project will begin in July of 2004.

References

American Association of Colleges of Nursing (1998). *The essentials of baccalaureate education for nursing practice.* Washington, DC: The American Association of Colleges of Nursing.

Baggett, LS (2001). Self-efficacy: Measurement and intervention in nursing. *Scholarly Inquiry for Nursing Practice,* 15(3) 183-188.

Bandura, A (1997). *Self efficacy: The exercise of control.* New York: WH Freeman & Co.

———. (ed.) (1995). *Self-efficacy in changing societies.* New York: Press Syndicate of the University of Cambridge.

———. (1989). Human agency in social cognitive theory. *American Psychologist,* 44, 1175-83.

———. (1986). *Social foundation of thought and action: A social cognitive theory.* Englewood Cliffs, NJ: Prentice-Hall, Inc.

———. (1982). A self-efficacy mechanism in human agency. *American Psychologist,* 37(2) 122-147.

———. (1977). *Social learning theory.* Englewood Cliffs, NJ: Prentice-Hall Inc.

Beck, AT (1972). *Depression: Causes and treatment.* Philadelphia: University of Pennsylvania Press.

Becker, H, Stuifbergen, A, Oh, H S & Hall, S (1993). Self-rated abilities for health practices: A health self-efficacy measure. *Health Values: Journal of Health Behavior, Education and Promotion,* 17(5) 42-50.

Campbell, JC (2002). Health consequences of intimate partner violence. *Lancet,* 359, 1331-36.

———, Jones, A-Snow, Dinemann, J, Kub, J, Schoelenberger, J, O'Campo, P, Gielen, A Carlson & Wynne, C (2002). Intimate partner violence and physical health consequences. *Archives of Internal Medicine,* 162, 1157-1163.

———, & Soeken, KL (1999). Women's responses to battering over time. *Journal of Interpersonal Violence,* 14(1) 21-40.

Coker, AL, Smith, PH, Bethea, L, King, MR & McKeown, RE (2000). Physical health consequences of physical and psychological intimate partner violence. *Archives of Family Medicine,* 9, 451-457.

Dutton, MA (1992). *Empowering and healing the battered woman.* New York: Springer Publishing Co.

Flaskerud, JH (1998). Vulnerable populations. In JJ Fitzpatrick (ed.). *Encyclopedia of nursing research.* New York: Springer.

Kolvenbach, PH (2000). The service of faith and the promotion of justice in American Jesuit higher education. Justice and Jesuit health sciences education. *Studies in the Spirituality of Jesuits,* 31(1) 1-29.

Lempert, LB (1996). Women's strategies for survival: Developing agency in abusive relationships. *Journal of Family Violence,* 11(3) 269-289.

Maibach, E & Murphy, DA (1995). Self-efficacy in health promotion research and practice: Conceptualization and measurement. *Health Education Research,* 10(1) 37-50.

Plichta, SB (1996). Violence and abuse: Implications for women's health. In MK Falik & KS Collins (eds). *Women's health, the commonwealth fund survey.* Baltimore, MD: The Johns Hopkins University Press.

Register, E (1993). Feminism and recovering from battering: Working with the individual women. In M Hansen & M Harway (eds.). Battering and family therapy: A feminist perspective. Newbury Park, CA: Sage.

Rodriguez, MA, Quiroga, S, Skupinki, S & Bauer, HM (1996). Breaking the silence: Battered women's perspectives on medical care. *Archives of Family Medicine,* 5, 153-158.

Sherer, M, Maddux, JE, Mercondante, B, Dunn, S, Prentice, Jacobs, B & Pregus, RW (1982). The Self-efficacy scale: Construction and validation. *Psychological Reports,* 5, 661-663.

Tyson, S & Fleming, B (1999). Conceptualizing battered women as a vulnerable population: A case study report. *Nursing Clinics of North America,* 34(2) 301-312.

Wood, G Goldberg & Middleman, RR (1992). Groups to empower battered women. *Journal of Women and Social Work,* 7(4) 82-96.

Yam, M (2000). Seen but not heard: Battered women's perceptions of the emergency department experience. *Journal of Emergency Nursing,* 26(5) 464-470.

16. Julie Sanford

Researching the Health Status of the Rural Caregiver

Conducting research in the area of rural health reflects our mission at Spring Hill College. Our mission statement says that, "We take the time and make the effort to teach and act with justice, with care and in service of others." Studying the problems of rural caregivers provides my students and me an opportunity to seek justice for some of America's most underserved and poor individuals.

The rural United States comprises 75% of the country's land and is home to 17% of the population. "Rural" is defined as places with fewer than 2,500 residents and open territory (United States Department of Agriculture Economic Research Service, 2003). Nurse practitioners tend to favor rural settings over urban areas; the number of nurse practitioners practicing in rural areas is 24.72 compared to urban rates of 20.08 per 100,000 of the population (Baer & Smith, 1999). But nurses are the exception among health care providers. For example, fewer than 9% of the nation's physicians are practicing in these areas even though 49 million Americans live in areas classified as rural (National Rural Health Association, 2003). The lack of access to health care professionals contributes to poorer health, higher mortality rates and greater morbidity rates from all causes among rural residents (Gamm et al., 2003).

The striking health disparity between urban and rural residents has been an important societal challenge for quite some time now. Ever more educational institutions try to prepare and motivate students for rural practice, and governmental agencies offer financial incentives to attract graduates to underserved rural areas e.g., educational loan forgiveness programs. The patients in rural areas are not the only ones who suffer disparities. Informal caregivers, that is, persons who provide direct support of patients with disabilities, usually at home, themselves suffer greater health risks (Agency for Healthcare Policy & Research, 1995).

Care giving can be stressful in any setting; however, the pressures that arise from access problems in the rural context can significantly exacerbate the stress on caregivers. There are additional factors to consider. Health agencies in these areas are less likely than are urban

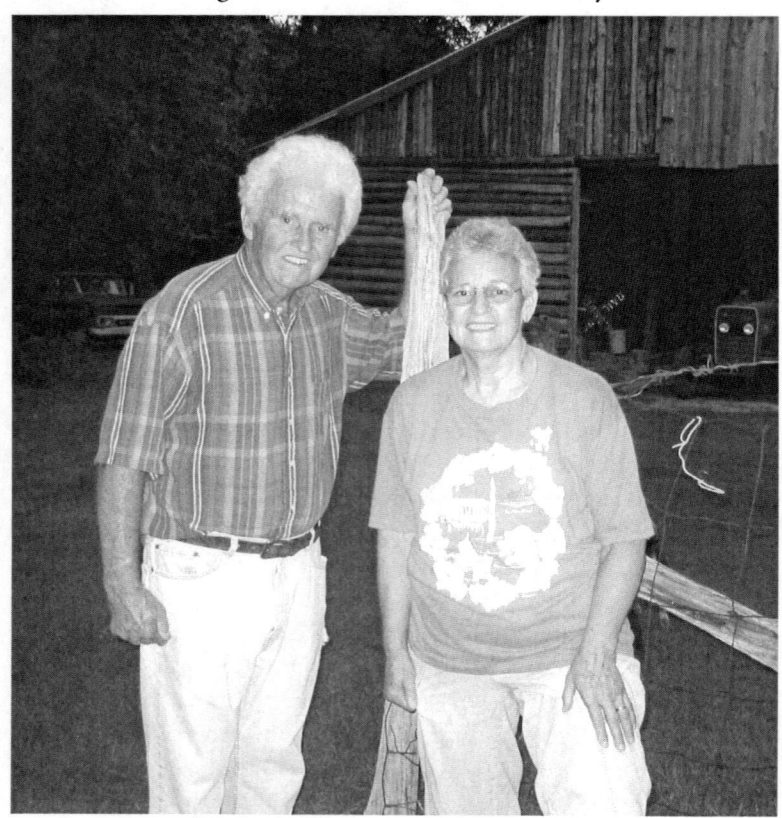

Rural Alabama resident Lena Tanner is the caregiver to her husband, Eugene Tanner, who suffers from Parkinson's Disease.
Photographer: Julie Sanford

agencies to be appropriately staffed and operated. They generally are smaller and offer fewer services (Cuellar & Butts, 1999). This patient population has higher rates of uninsured patients than does the urban population. The larger proportion of small businesses and lower paying jobs makes it less likely that residents will have employer-supported health insurance (Gamm et al., 2003). In addition, rural home health care agencies have been especially harmed by the recent more stringent reimbursement rules adopted by Medicare, the national system that covers the oldest US citizens. The net result of all of these factors is that rural caregivers are under a great burden when providing care to their loved ones. Feelings of stress, burden and worries about their own health can in fact become overwhelming.

Much has been written about the care giving experience. In spite of the challenges that rural caregivers face, it remains an understudied area. I first became interested in rural care giving when completing the clinical experience for my doctoral studies. I noted that though hospitalized patients were receiving excellent physical care, their caregivers were anxious, stressed and expressed feelings of fear. When spending time with a home health nurse, I found that rural caregivers talked about social isolation and complained of not being able to care for their own health.

My study* explored the relationships among stress, caregiver burden and the health status of rural caregivers. I used a descriptive-correlational design to explore the caregiver health status of 63 informal caregivers in rural Alabama and Mississippi. The research confirmed that burden and stress are significant predictors of the health status of these caregivers. They complained of uncomfortable physical symptoms, reported their health to be much poorer than that of the general population, and experienced difficulty with transportation to the hospital and their physicians.

My initial study was followed by interviews of rural caregivers, funded in part by a Teagle Faculty Development grant. The primary objective of the qualitative study was to hear the caregivers' words about how they see the relationship between care giving and their own health. What have been their experiences in caring for family members? What interventions do they see as helping to decrease their stress and burden? What common physical health problems do they experience? I interviewed eight rural caregivers. The interviews were transcribed and analyzed using analysis techniques. Several themes emerged from the data including: (1) social isolation; (2) going to the doctor; (3) health activities; (4) distance; (5) neglected health; (6) health diagnoses; (7) worry about future; (8) social support; (9) worry about leaving the care recipient.

Upon publication of the results, I hope to apply for external funding for an interventional study that may decrease burden and stress and improve the morbidity and mortality rates of informal rural caregivers. In the mean time, our Spring Hill College nursing students benefit from exposure to these and other societal issues related to care giving. Our future graduates will be working closely with informal caregivers in many different settings. Nurses must learn how their rural patients will be cared for at home, what problems must be anticipated and what difficulties informal caregivers experience.

At our Jesuit colleges and universities, we must do more than simply study the injustices of the health disparities between America's rural and urban health care systems. We are under a moral obligation to address injustice as best we know how. My journey in the area of rural care giving health is one that I hope will ultimately result in improving health outcomes for those rural Americans overwhelmed with the demands of providing care to their chronically ill family members.

* Partial findings from this study can be found in Sanford, J & Townsend-Rocchiccioli, J (2004). The perceived health status of rural caregivers. *Geriatric Nursing, 25*(3), 145-148.

References

Agency for Health Care Policy and Research. (1995). *Clinical practice guideline: Post-stroke rehabilitation.* Washington, DC: US Department of Health and Human Services.

Baer, L & Smith, L (1999). Non-physician professionals and rural America. In TC Ricketts (ed.). *Rural health in the United States.* New York, NY: Oxford University Press.

Cuellar, N & Butts, J (1999). Caregiver distress: What nurses in rural settings can do to help. *Nursing Forum,* 34(3) 24-30.

Gamm, L, Hutchison, L, Dabney, B, & Dorsey, A, (eds.). (2003). Rural healthy people 2010: A companion document to healthy people 2010. Volume 2. College Station, Texas: The Texas A & M University System

Health Science Center. http://www.srph.tamushsc.edu/centers/rhp2010/index.html (site accessed 7/22/04).

National Rural Health Association (2003). *Rural graduate medical education.* http://www.nrharural.org/pagefile/issuepapers/ipaper22.html (site accessed 7/22/04).

Sanford, J, & Townsend-Rocchiccioli, J, (2004). The perceived health status of rural caregivers. *Geriatric Nursing*, 25(3) 145-148.

United States Department of Agriculture Economic Research Service (2003). *Key topics: Rural America.* Retrieved http://www.ers.usda.gov/Topics/view.asp?T=104000 (site accessed 7/22/04).

Part IV

Administrative Commentaries

17. Fortunato Cristobal

Toward Unity for Health in Medical Education: A Case from the Philippines

I. Health in our Region

Nearly one third of the Philippines' 72 million people live on Mindanao Island. Zamboanga City (population 0.6 million) is the hub for services in Western Mindanao and the Sulu Archipelago (population 3.6 million), one of the most medically underserved areas of the south Pacific. Seventy percent of the people live in rural densely populated shorelines of the islands. Travel is predominantly by boat, access to inland areas is mostly by foot.

Health problems abound. Neonatal tetanus, measles, typhoid, cholera, dengue fever, tuberculosis, malaria, diarrhea and respiratory infections are major problems in these areas. The fertility rate is about five children for each woman, and infant mortality is more than 75 deaths per 1000 births. Safe water, balanced nutrition, prenatal care and full immunization remain long term health goals. There are 28 medical schools in the Philippines but none in this region, and few physicians are willing to move to this underdeveloped area.

II. Planning a Medical School for Unity of Health and Development

Against this background and aware of the challenge of starting a new school with very limited resources, we initiated consultations between the community, health professionals and academic stakeholders. As a result of the meetings, participants proposed a new, private, not-for-profit medical school. The school was to be a collaborative effort between several groups. The Jesuit university, Ateneo de Zamboanga, would provide teaching facilities such as library and modular rooms; the local doctors would volunteer as faculty; patients from the community would provide experiential learning to the students as well as some of the students themselves; local businessmen would raise funds; and the local Health Department would provide financial assistance for research. A board of fifteen members composed of three academicians, five civic leaders and seven doctors formed an oversight and governance group.

Our next task was to develop an educational program for selecting and training a new kind of professional who would be proficient in managing disease and competent to improve the public health. We contacted leaders in medical education at the World Health Organization (WHO) including experts from the UK, the USA, Canada, New Zealand and the Philippines.

Our emphasis was to be on public health problems. Most medical schools work with patients suffering from complex medical problems and they prepare students to be specialists for practice in hospitals in urban centers. Their training mostly ignores disease prevention, health promotion, community development and the social and economic determinants of health. Since we could not find a model that was ideally suited to our situation, we created one.

III. The Beginnings—Vision and Mission

In 1993, we held weekend development seminars for volunteer faculty to discuss the psychology of learning, problem solving, new methods of evaluating students and curriculum design. The school opened in June 1994, and since then students and faculty have worked together to modified our new programs. Mentors from Canada and New Zealand assisted with the faculty development, curriculum planning and learning experiences.

The vision of the dean and board of trustees is incorporated into the Vision Statement of the Zamboanga Medical School Foundation (ZMSF):

The ZMSF envisions the medical school to pioneer and implement a curriculum that combines competence and problem-based instruction with experiential learning in the community, that is responsive to the changing patterns of health care development and the needs of these communities and is sensitive to the social and cultural realities of Western Mindanao.

The mission of our school is simply stated: "The medical school exists to help provide solutions to the health problems of the people and communities of Western Mindanao. . . ."

Piece by piece we developed an integrated curriculum with problem-based learning, community-oriented and community-based education and competency-based evaluations. All basic science and clinical learning is integrated into the problem-based approach. Three educational strands are intertwined: a working problem strand, a population strand and a professional skills strand.

As we progressed, four additional dimensions became central in our planning:

Faculty Development. We recognized the need to train our faculty— graduates of traditional medical schools—with the tools for this new curriculum. This requirement led to a faculty development program with the option of earning a Masters of Medical Educational degree.

Career Options. Our students needed a career option for medical specialties that could equip and qualify them for field positions in the Department of Health. This need led to an optional Master of Public Health tract for the fifth (first post graduate) year of the program. This MD-MPH has also become attractive to some members of faculty.

CME of Graduates. A survey among the alumni disclosed the concern and need for continuing medical education (CME) that resulted from geographical isolation. To address these issues, we introduced the alternative residency training program in family medicine. This program will provide the linkage for referral/consultations and the continuing medical education for our graduates through distance learning. While they retain their post in the community, they can earn specialty units through this program to qualify them for the family medicine specialty board examination so that they can eventually become family medicine specialists.

Scholarship Grant. Our students do not come from the upper economic strata of the Philippine society. Those who can afford to do so choose to study medicine in the major institutions of Manila and Cebu. We are therefore confronted with the need to support students who are academically capable to study medicine but are economically disadvantaged. The school has embarked on scholarship grants that pay for their tuition. However, upon graduation the recipients are obliged to return service by committing to practice medicine in the region for a time equivalent to the years of their scholarship grant. Currently, 60% of our student population are on full educational grants.

We enroll about 15-35 students each year depending on the qualification of the applicants. Over the last ten years, we have graduated 71 students from our program—26 of them with MD/MPH degrees. Fifty-five of them have passed the national medical licensing board examination and are now occupying medical positions in distant communities once considered doctorless areas. Equipped in skills of community development, these medical missionaries are affecting changes in the remote communities of this region.

18. André Piront, SJ

Forming Future Physicians: A Report from Belgium

In the anatomy class room, our third year medical students learn concretely a lesson that is of great importance to their future work. This lesson comes as they are dissecting the bodies of deceased persons who have agreed to serve yet beyond their own death toward the formation of future medical doctors and through them, the well-being of future patients. On a wall of this class room, a Latin sentence reads: *Et expecto resurrectionem mortuorum*—"And I expect the resurrection of the dead."

This sentence is taken from the Christian creed, and one may wonder why it is written in this place. Evidently it would not be there if the medical school was not Christian. The sign does not command much attention and anyone who notices it may pass it by without really paying attention to it. But if the passerby stops to think for a moment, the question of why the quotation is there will surface. Maybe those who do notice will come to see differently the bodies they are so closely observing as they learn anatomy. Will they recall the mystery of death that is open to hope for believers?

This local feature shows why the Facultés Universitaires Notre-Dame de la Paix in Namur, Belgium, have a medical school. This university was founded by the Society of Jesus. It has inherited values from a humanist and Jesuit tradition. It draws on this tradition for inspiration and the interpretation of its missions of teaching, research and service to the community.

Our school of medicine contributes to the formation of future medical doctors. They will devote themselves to those who are suffering, believing that all human beings are of extraordinary value, regardless of their age, their condition, their social state, their way of life. This belief is an act of faith that is shared by physicians in general around the world. The Christian message strengthens this manner of seeing this profession, because illness and handicap do not alter human dignity.

Our school of medicine must complete its educational mission in a limited number of years, because it does not offer a full curriculum. In order to complete their medical education, after three years in Namur the students must transfer to one of the other Belgian medical schools that offer a complete curriculum, including hospital rotations. We have learned that those schools greatly appreciate our preparatory curriculum. During the three years the students study with us, we achieve many things. We provide the students with a scientific basis that prepares them to fulfill their clinical duties and enables them to perform a good diagnostic exam. In order to do this successfully, students must acquire much scientific knowledge and the ability to think with precision and integrity. But a good physician must also be able to maintain a good rapport with those he or she helps. Physicians must attain a sense of social responsibility. Their scientific formation must be in harmony with human value. Hence, our medical curriculum includes courses in philosophy, ethics, psychology and religious sciences. In order to promote students' humanistic development, we facilitate ample contact between teachers and students.

Located in a well-developed country, our school of medicine has established exchanges with other medical schools in the developing world, for example, Benin, Congo, Liban, Madagascar, Ruanda and Vietnam. We share certain pedagogical documents, using video or multimedia tools, and we welcome foreign scientists.

Our school also maintains a research program including amongst other issues, research on subcellular structures and membrane traffic in normal and pathological conditions; keratinocyte differentiation; the role of the renal inner medulla and electrolyte homeostasis in the genesis of arterial hypertension; and the function of the MAGE proteins in the mouse. We collaborate with several organizations that are concerned with the use of rehabilitation technologies by the disabled. Thus, through its laboratories, the school tries to contribute to the progression of human knowledge and understanding.

Among the five medical schools in the French-speaking part of Belgium, Namur stands out. Students come here because they know

Forming Future Physicians: A Report from Belgium

they will receive a strong yet distinct formation, as well as the help needed to fulfill these goals. When they leave Namur to continue their medical studies elsewhere, they exhibit competency but also witness to the importance of human relating that has helped them achieve that competency during their tenure with us. May they also preserve faith in humankind and belief in the dignity of each person.

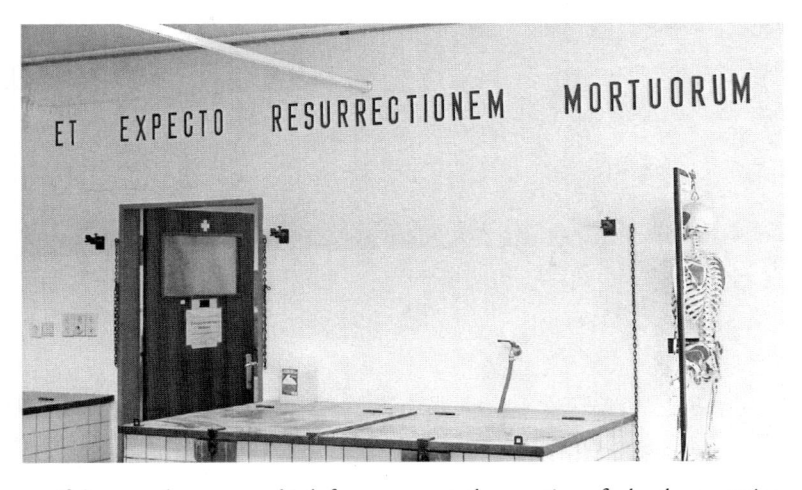

... if the passerby stops to think for a moment, the question of why the quotation is there will surface. Maybe those who do notice will come to see differently the bodies they are so closely observing as they learn anatomy.
Photographer: Jos VM Welie

19. F. Daniel Davis

The Jesuit Medical School & its Leadership Role in Healing Medical Education

I had not seen KB for several months. She was one of the first students I had met and come to know after moving into my position as a curriculum dean and faculty member at Georgetown's School of Medicine. At that time, she was a first-year medical student whose character and sense of purpose seemed to me to reflect the ideal physician-in-formation: she was bright and engaging, honest and caring and animated by a commitment to the "good"—the good of her future patients and the broader "social good." The graduate of a well-known Catholic college, KB had been drawn to Georgetown by its Jesuit identity and values, particularly by the emphasis placed on *cura personalis*—the care of the (whole) person. During her first and then her second year of medical school, she was a frequent visitor to my office where we talked about the challenges and the stresses of being a medical student. Now in the midst of her third year, when clinical rotations often take students to hospitals throughout metropolitan Washington, she and I had had little contact.

And so it was that I was happy that day to hear a knock at my door, open it and find KB standing there. She stood there however, with a look of obvious distress on her face and quietly asked if we could talk. I welcomed her into my office, she sat down and as she began to speak, tears filled her eyes and she bowed her head low. My mind raced through possible explanations for her distress while I extended a hand to comfort her, to help her compose herself and her thoughts. After a few minutes of sitting there in silence, she began to speak. "I do not like the person I am becoming. And yet I feel that I have no choice. If I want to be a doctor, I have to become what they want me to be. But I don't want to be that kind of doctor. I think I would rather quit first. . . ."

I was not unaware of the phenomenon emerging before my eyes that day in the office with KB. I had worked in academic medicine for fifteen years and had, through my studies and work in clinical ethics, become familiar with the issues and problems characteristic of the ethical formation of physicians. One such issue or problem has been repeatedly reported in the literature: that is, the tendency of physicians to become more cynical in the course of their education and training. In their often cited study, Feudtner, Christakis and Christakis (1994) describe a related phenomenon as "ethical erosion" and detail their observations of this phenomenon among a cohort of medical students.

In my relatively brief time in a decanal job, however, I had not encountered these phenomena so directly and in such a poignant fashion as I did that day with KB. Here was a student who embodied the idealism that often animates our vision of what physicians can and should be: healers whose advanced knowledge and technical skill are exceeded only by their compassion and dedication to the care of the vulnerable and sick. The distress that she voiced to me that day was distress in the face of what she perceived to be an institutionalized abandonment of that very idealism. She saw an abandonment operationalized in a pervasive effort to transform individuals who are drawn to medicine by visions of helping and healing into technically proficient body mechanics, devoid of feelings or values that interfere with efficient "management" of patient problems. The "they" to whom she referred were the residents and the attending physicians whose behaviors—with patients, with each other and with students—are perhaps the most critically decisive factor in the learning process of the clinical years. Although there were exceptions, she explained, most seemed determined to "hammer" her into an exact replica of themselves—preoccupied with objective data and information; concerned only tangentially, if at all, with the individuals in their care; harried and exhausted by an unceasingly furious pace; driven by considerations of cost and efficiency.

Often, when she raised broader concerns about her patients—what would happen to them after they are discharged? could they care for themselves? what significance does this illness have for their families, for their sense of their own future—she was abruptly "brought up short" and advised to "focus on what is really important here"—the pathophysiology, the diagnosis, the technical management challenges of this or that disease. "I know these are all essential," she explained, "but I deliberately chose to come to Georgetown, because I thought—I was told that it is—a place that values the patient in a fundamental way—that practices humanism and doesn't just pay it lip service."

Over the past six years, I've had more opportunities to explore the gap into which KB had fallen—the gap between the "real" and the "ideal" in medicine and medical education. It is from the vantage point of this experience—flawed and limited to be sure—that I take up the question of the mission of Jesuit institutions in health professional education, particularly Jesuit medical schools. Is their mission different from the missions of other institutions, that is, of a secular or otherwise religious orientation? If the mission of a Jesuit medical school is different, how is it so? We can gain a foothold on the complexities of this question by considering that every medical school engages in the education and training of future members of a *profession*. In its most originary sense, a profession is a collective of individuals whose identity rests on the shared promise to help other human beings who experience some fundamental human need—in the case of physicians and other health professionals, the need for healing. Physicians are educated and trained to make good on this promise. Indeed, their keeping the promise at the core of their identities is contingent upon their mastery of scientific knowledge and technical skill. Fidelity to the promise is also based on the physician's continual cultivation and demonstration of a set of interrelated virtues critical to healing in the broadest sense of the word. By "virtues" I mean such habitual predispositions as honesty, integrity, trustworthiness, compassion and empathy, temperance, justice and of special relevance to this exchange, altruism. Thus we could argue that the mission of *every* medical school is to ensure that its future physicians are, through their acquired knowledge, skill and virtue, fit to keep the promise that defines the profession. In other words, in light of this shared mission, there is no basis for differentiating the Jesuit from the secular or from the otherwise religious, medical school.

How effectively are medical schools fulfilling this mission? The data to which we might turn in answering this question are far flung, fragmentary and variable. An authentically scholarly treatment of the question would require a much more methodic and systematic analysis of information and data regarding for example, patient satisfaction, mortality and morbidity, etc. Instead, I believe we can get at least a provocative proxy answer to the question if we note first, that for the last 20 years American medical education has sounded a fairly steady drum beat for change prompted by the perception that something is amiss in the way we educate future physicians: that not only are our pedagogies and assessment methods inadequate to the challenges of educating professionals, the very culture of medicine and medical education can be inimical to the ideals to which the profession has long laid claim. The pedagogical emphasis on didactic lectures, rote memorization of biomedical facts and passive learning; the lack of integration among basic and clinical disciplines in the teaching and learning process; the bias-inflected methods in the assessment of clinical competence; the relative neglect of effective values-based learning and professional formation—numerous panels of "experts" have repeatedly diagnosed these and other defects in medical education that in large measure continue to await successful therapy.

Complicating this situation are two complex forces. One encompasses all the factors that relate to the evolving organization, delivery and financing of health care. These factors have particular importance in health care delivered by academic health centers, which have experienced profound institutional stress in the last two decades or so. These are factors that are reshaping medical education for good as well as ill. The other force has to do with the culture of medicine, which also presents a mix of salutary and malignant features for the mission of professional formation. Among the more malignant features are the often obsequious deference to hierarchy, the cult of technical expertise, the devaluation of feeling and affect and the tendency to promote the self-interest of physicians at the expense of altruism.

Indeed, one of the more rueful conclusions that I have reached in the last several years is this: medical students are subject to a barrage of incentives that encourage and promote self-interest such that it is remarkable that any emerge from the educational process with an intact sense of altruism. I know that many leave medical school with a deeply felt commitment to the welfare of others, but I am often inclined to the view that they do so despite, rather than because of, the educational process. It is in this context, subject as it is to these forces, that medical students forge their identity as health care professionals.

If my admittedly rather bleak perspective on the efficacy of the mission of professional formation is nonetheless somewhat accurate, what then is the role of the Jesuit medical school? Specifically, what role can or perhaps should it play in healing medical education? I believe that role is nothing less than that of leading the efforts that are now underway to effect another far-reaching reform of physician education—particularly in the arena of values-based professional formation. Jesuit institutions are I believe unique in their explicit, persistent commitment to the values of integrative care of the whole person—of *cura personalis*. They work from a still viable tradition of education rooted in the notion of shaping young men and women "for others." They have, as a critical resource of institutional conscience, this commitment and this tradition. How can they ensure that this commitment and this tradition "live" and are visibly present in the formal and the hidden curriculum? I offer the following suggestions as concrete examples for operationalizing the values of Jesuit education.

• First, in their admissions policies, in addition to emphasizing grade point averages and MCAT scores, they should emphasize—even require—experience in community service and evidence of the clinical virtues critical to clinical "competence," with "competence" understood in the broadest, most holistic sense possible.

• Second, they should promote the teaching, learning and assessment of these virtues as strenuously as they do scientific/clinical knowledge and technical skill.

• Third, the success of this second initiative depends upon the institution's will to hold faculty responsible and accountable for effective role-modeling of these same virtues. Without such responsibility and accountability, all talk of inculcating virtue among students is just that—talk.

• Fourth, learning in the context of service, particularly service to the disadvantaged, should also be required, preferably as a longitudinal experience beginning with the first and running through the fourth year of medical school.

- Fifth, promotion and graduation should be as dependent upon a student's demonstration of altruism and the other clinical virtues as it now is upon success with the board exams and other traditional measures.

None of these is an original proposal. In one form or the other each can be found among the now thousands of recommendations for change emanating from the numerous expert panels that have sought to address the contemporary ills of medical education. There remains, however, the unrealized potential for originality in leading the effort to implement, rigorously and effectively, these much needed therapies for healing medical education. Jesuit medical schools should—and indeed must—seize and act upon this potential, if only in fulfillment of the obligation we have to the many students who, like KB, believe that we not only espouse but also practice our values.

Reference

1994. Feudtner, C, Christakis, D & Christakis, N. Do clinical clerks suffer ethical erosion? Students' perceptions of their ethical environment and personal development. Academic Medicine, 69, 670-679.

Part V

Appendices

20. *Documents on Jesuit Health Care & Health Sciences Education*

Diccionario de Historia de la Compania de Jesús, Vol 1-4. Madrid-Roma 2001.
  Contains several articles on the involvement of Jesuits in health care, including
  Farmacias (Anagnostou, S & McNaspy, CJ, 1377-1379)
  Medicina (Ziggelaar, A & McNaspy, CJ, 2601-2602)
  Psicología (Royce, JE, 3250-3253)
  Psiquiatría y Psichoterapia (Meisner, WW, 3253-3256)

Andrade, B (1994). Towards an Ignatian understanding of suffering. Review of Ignatian spirituality. (CIS) XXV 3(77) 46-62.

Baldwin, M (1993). Alchemy and the Society of Jesus in the seventeenth century: Strange bedfellows. *Ambix* 40(2) 41-64.

Bajaen, EM (1995). Sex, moral and medicine in counter reformation Spain. An unpublished report on pollution by the Jesuit Miguel Perex (1550-1605). *Dynamis*, 15, 443-457.

Barr, WG (1996). Jesuit medical schools: Enriching US health care. *America*, 175(15) 6-9.

Baumiller, RC (1999) On being a medical geneticist in the post-GC 34 era. In Tripole, M (1999). *Promise renewed: Jesuit higher education for a new millennium*. Chicago: Jesuit Way.

———. (1998). Companions in health care transitions. Paper presented at the National Jesuit Health Care Conference, Boston, MA.

Bieri, JW (1954). The training of a doctor. *Jesuit Educational Quarterly*, 16, 223-239.

Blum, PR (2001). The Jesuits and the Janus faced history of natural sciences. In J Helm & A. Winkelman (eds.). *Religious confessions and the sciences in the 16th century*. Leiden/Boston: Brill.

Burghardt, W (1995). Biblical justice and "the cry of the poor": Jesuit medicine and the third millennium. In M Huey (ed.). (1994). *Caring for the body, the mind and the soul. Vol. 1: The Jesuit tradition and medicine* Washington, DC: Georgetown University (reprinted in this volume).

Calverley, RK (1980). St. René: The patron saint of aneasthesists and a patron saint of Canada. *Canad. Anesth. Soc. J.*, 27(1) 74-77.

Cassmen, E (1995). Stethoscope for divine murmurs: Modern psychiatry and the Jesuits. In M Huey (ed.). (1994). *Caring for the body, the mind and the soul. Vol. 1: The Jesuit tradition and medicine* Washington, DC: Georgetown University.

Charles P (1935) *Les anciens jésuites et la médecine en Chine.* Xaveriana, Vol. 135. Louvain: Museum Lessianum Louvain.

Curran, E (1995). The Jesuit tradition and the first hundred years of medicine at Georgetown from "sundown college" to medical center. In M Huey (ed.). (1994). *Caring for the body, the mind and the soul. Vol. 1: The Jesuit tradition and medicine* Washington, DC: Georgetown University.

Daxecker, F (2000). Der Jesuit Athanasius Kirchner und sein Organum mathematicum. *Gesnerus,* 57(1-2) 77-83.

del Rio, ME & Revuelta, M (1995). Enfermerías y boticas en las casas de la Compagñía en Madrid, siglio XVI-XIX. *AHSI,* 64, 39-81.

Delattre, P (1934). Un institut de médecine des missions au Japon au XVI siècle. *RHM,* 11, 16-28.

Desmet, M (1996/1998*). Dag en nacht. een spiritualiteit van de medische ervaring.* Tielt: Lannoo.

Drane, JK (1951). Content of medical college admission test. *Jesuit Educational Quarterly,* 13, 185-187.

Ferrari, A (1956). Il controbuto dei gesuiti allo sviluppo della medicina nel IV centenario della morte di S. Ignazio di Loyola (1556-1956). *Minerva Medica II,* varia 528-552

Fodstad H (2002). et al. Barbarian medicine in feudal Japan [with commentaries]. *Neurosurgery,* 51(4) 1015-1025.

Garraghan, GJ (1938). The Jesuits of the middle United States. New York: America Press. Contains information about founding of US medical schools.

Gicklhorn, R (1973). *Missionsapoteker. Deuthsche Pharmazenten in Lateinamerika des 17. und 18. Jahrhts.* Stuttgart.

Gilroy, J (1956). Ignatian heritage: Jesuits and medicine. *Linacre Quarterly,* 23, 56-559.

Goodier, A (1931). Jesuit's bark. *Month,* 157, 97-106.

Guerino AA (1986). Herman medical Jesuits in America. In *XXX Congrès Internationale d'Histoire de Médecine, Actes* (1988). Duesseldorf, 875-878.

Guerrero, G (1997). Salud y enfermedad en Ignacio de Loyola. Aspectos biográficos. *Anuario Instituto Ignacio de Loyola,* 4, 115-128.

Guthrie, H (1943). Catholic emphasis and influence in our graduate and professional schools. *Jesuit Educational Quarterly,* VI, 40-41.

Gysel, C (1989). L'Encyclopedie d'Etienne Binet (1621), La médicine et l'odontologie. *Rev. Odontostomatologie (Paris),* 18(6) 497-504.

Hahn, K, Radded, JM, Fellers, JE (2001). Spiritual care: Bridging the disciplines in congregational health ministries. *Journal of Health Care Chaplaincy,* 11(2) 49-60.

Harney, MP (1962). *The Jesuit in history. The Society of Jesus through four centuries.* Chicago: Loyola University Press.

Harris SJ (1996). Confession building, long-distance networks, and the organization of Jesuit science. *Early Science and Medicine,* 1(3) 287-318.

Heinrich, K & Walter, C. (1995). Ignatius von Loyola - genial oder psychisch krank? *Fortscr. Neurol. Psychiat.,* 63, 213-219.

Hrubetz, J (1993). Nursing education in Jesuit universities and colleges. The art of science and caring. *Conversations,* Spring, 18-19.

M Huey, (ed.). (1994). *Caring for the body, the mind and the soul. Vol. 1: The Jesuit tradition and medicine.* Washington, DC: Georgetown University.

Ignatius T (1985). Francisco de Borja, Duke of Gandia - On prayer and penance. In JN Tylenda (ed. and trans.). (1985). *Saint Ignatius Loyola: Counsels for Jesuits.* Selected letters and instructions. Chicago: Loyola University Press, 30-33.

———. (1985). Father Antonio Araoz - On caring for one's health. In JN Tylenda (ed. and trans.). (1985). *Saint Ignatius Loyola: Counsels for Jesuits.* Selected letters and instructions. Chicago: Loyola University Press, 47-48.

———. (1985). Teutonio da Braganca - On sickness as an excercise of virtue. In JN Tylenda (ed. and trans.). (1985). *Saint Ignatius Loyola: Counsels for Jesuits.* Selected letters and instructions. Chicago: Loyola University Press, 87-89.

———. (1985). Father Gaspar Berze - On moderation in penance. In JN Tylenda (ed. and trans.). (1985). *Saint Ignatius Loyola: Counsels for Jesuits.* Selected letters and instructions. Chicago: Loyola University Press, 91-93.

———. (1985). Francesco de Attino - On preserving one's health for God's service. In JN Tylenda (ed. and trans.). (1985). *Saint Ignatius Loyola: Counsels for Jesuits.* Selected letters and instructions. Chicago: Loyola University Press, 94-95.

Jaramillo-Arango, J (1946-52). A critical review of the basic facts in the history of Cinchona. *Journal of the Linnean Society of London, Botany,* 53, 272-309.

Jarrett, S (2003). Where loyalties lie. *Conversations on Jesuit Higher Education,* Fall, 24, 44-45.

Laforet, EG (1957). De militis magni corpore. Being an account of the medical history: Death and necropsy in the case of the venerable Ignatius of Loyola (1491-1556), general of the Company of Jesus. *Linacre Quarterly,* 24, 85-89.

Lombillo, JR (1973). The soldier saint—a psychological analysis of the conversion of Ignatius of Loyola. *Psych. Q.,* 47(3) 386-418.

Lutterbach, H (1994). 'Auf die Krafte des Leibes achten!' Die Bedeutung der Gesundheit im Leben und Wirken des Ignatius von Loyola. *Theologie und Philosophie,* 69, 556-569.

Martin, AL (1988). *The Jesuit mind: the mentality of an elite in early modern France.* Ithaca: Cornell University Press.

———. (1996). *Plague? Jesuit accounts of epidemic disease in the 16th century.* Kirksville: Sixteenth Century Journal Publishers.

McGrath, E (1960). Liberal education in the professions. *Jesuit Educational Quarterly,* 22, 197-200.

Meissner, WW (1999*). To the greater glory - a psychological study of Ignatian spirituality.* Milwaukee, WI: Marquette University Press.

O'Brien, RL (2002). Why does Creighton have a medical center? *Creighton University Magazine,* Fall, 55.

O'Connell, LJ (1988). The preferential options for the poor and health care in the United States. In Monagle, JF & Thomasma DC (1993). *Medical ethics: A guide for health professionals.* Rockville: Apsen Publishers, ch. 26, 306-313.

O'Donovan, L (2002). For the most high cometh healing. Festvortrag zum fünfjährigen Bestehen des Unfallkrankhaus Berlin (unpublished lecture).

O'Malley, JW (1993). *The first Jesuits.* Cambridge: Harvard University Press.

Padberg, SJ, J (1993). The Jesuit tradition and medicine. Unpublished lecture. The Jesuit Vision and Heritage Seminar, Loyola University Medical Center, Chicago, Jan 20.

The sources of the Jesuit tradition a history for the future. In M Huey (ed.). (1994). *Caring for the body, the mind and the soul. Vol. 1: The Jesuit tradition and medicine.* Washington, DC: Georgetown University

Quintal, J (1995). René Goupil: Patron saint of anesthetists. *Journal of the American Association of Nurse Anesthetists,* 63(3) 191-193.

Radde, JM (1984). Spiritual needs assessment tool. *Journal of Christian Healing,* 6(2) 17-18.

———. (1987). Wounded healers? *Journal of Christian Healing,* 9(2) 48.

———. (1984). Preparing to give spiritual care. *Journal of Christian Healing,* 6(2) 15-16.

Rahner, H (1955-56). Der kranke Ignatius. *Stimmen der Zeit,* 158, 81-90.
——— (1946-47). Die Granschrift des Loyola. *Stimmen der Zeit,* 139, 321-337.
Rompel, J (1929). Der Arzt Baldo und die Chinarinde. *Stimmer der Zeit,* 117, 124-136.
Rosenman, LD (1996) Fact and fiction: The death of Saint Ignatius of Loyola. *Surgery,* 119,1 56-60. (See also commentary by Flaherty and response by Rosenman, *Surgery* 120(5) 903-904).
Schwitalla, A (1954). The medical apostolate of the American assistancy. *Woodstock Letters,* 83, 227-300.
———. (1940). Early Jesuit writings on medicine. A note on the Jesuit quadricentennial. *Hospital Progress,* 21, 389-392.
Sheehan, M. Medicine as ministry, with thanks and hope: celebrating 450 years of Jesuit heritage. Chicago: The Jesuit Community Corp. at Loyola University,
Shoup, G, (1971). What kind of a human being should we let scientists make in their labs? In Riemer, G (1971). *The new Jesuits.* Boston: Little, Brown & Co.
Teixeira, M (1970). Luis de Almeida (+1583), médico, comerciante e missionário. *BEDMA,* 68, 521-582.
Treutlein, ThE (1940). The Jesuit missionary in the role of the physician. *Mid-America,* 22, 120-141.
Valverde, JL (1978). *Presencia de la Compagñía de Jesús en el desarrollo de la Farmacia.* Granada.
Waardt, H (1996). Chasing demons and curing mortals: The medical practice of clerics in the Netherlands. In H Marland & M Pelling (eds.). *The task of healing. Medicine, religion and gender in England and the Netherlands 1450-1800.* Rotterdam: Erasmus Publishing, 171-203.
Weigel, G (1929). The society and the lepers. *Woodstock Letters,* 58, 347-350.
Welie, JVM (2003). Saint Ignatius' attitude towards the body, health and health care. *National Catholic Bioethics Quarterly,* 3(2) 247-255.
——— (2003) Ignatius of Loyola on medical education. Or should today's Jesuits continue to run health sciences schools? *Early Science and Medicine,* 8(1) 26-43.
Wickham, J (1954). The worldly ideal of Inigo Loyola. *Thought,* 29, 209-236.
Ziller, C (2001). Jesuits and alchemy in the early seventeenth century: Father Johannes Roberti and the weapon-salve controversy. *Ambix,* 48(2) 83-101.

21. Contributors

Frank Ayers, DDS
Associate Dean for Student Affairs and Director of Admissions
School of Dentistry
Creighton University Medical Center
Omaha, Nebraska, USA
fayers@creighton.edu

Frank Bernt, PhD
Associate Professor, Health Services Department
Director, Faith-Justice Institute
St. Joseph University
Philadelphia, Pennsylvania, USA
fbernt@sju.edu

Rachel Bognet
University of Scranton
Philadelphia
Scranton, Pennsylvania, USA
bognetr2@UofS.edu

Walter Burghardt, SJ
Professor Emeritus, Theology, Catholic University of America
Provincial Residence
Baltimore, Maryland, USA
wburghardt@loyola.edu

Peter Clark, SJ, PhD
Associate Professor of Theology
Director, Health Care Ethics Program
St. Joseph University
Philadelphia, Pennsylvania, USA
pclark@sju.edu

Fortunato Cristobal, MD
Founding Dean
Zamboanga Medical School Foundation
Zamboanga City, Philippines
president@central.adzu.edu.ph

F. Daniel Davis, PhD
Associate Dean
Educational Planning and Evaluation
Georgetown University School of Medicine
Washington, DC, USA
davisd@georgetown.edu

Rosanna F. DeMarco, PhD, APRN,BC, ACRN
William F. Connell School of Nursing
Boston College
Boston, Massachusetts, USA
RDema10519@aol.com

Judith Lee Kissell, PhD
Assistant Professor
Center for Health Policy and Ethics
Creighton University Medical Center
Omaha, Nebraska, USA
jkissell@creighton.edu

Peter-Hans Kolvenbach, SJ
Superior General
Society of Jesus
Rome, Italy

Thomas Massaro, SJ, PhD
Associate Professor
Weston Jesuit School of Theology
Cambridge, Massachusetts, USA
tmassaro@wjst.edu

Anne E. Norris, PhD, APRN,BC, FAAN
William F. Connell School of Nursing
Boston College
Boston, Massachusetts, USA
anne.norris.1@bc.edu

Kirk Peck, PT, MS, CSCS
Assistant Professor
Department of Physical Therapy
Creighton University Medical Center
Omaha, Nebraska, USA
kpeck@creighton.edu

André Piront, SJ, MD
Professor of General Physiology.
Faculty of Medicine
Facultés Universitaires Notre-Dame de la Paix
Namur, Belgium
andre.piront@fundp.ac.be

Julie Sanford, DNS, RN
Assistant Professor of Nursing
Spring Hill College
Mobile, Alabama
jsanford@shc.edu

Miriam Schulman
Communications Director
Markkula Center for Applied Ethics
Santa Clara University
Santa Clara, CA, USA
mschulman@scu.edu

William E. Stempsey, SJ, MD, PhD
Associate Professor
Department of Philosophy
College of the Holy Cross
Worcester, Massachusetts, USA
wstempsey@holycross.edu

Jos VM Welie, MMedS, JD, PhD
Professor
Center for Health Policy and Ethics
& Department of Community and Preventive Dentistry
Creighton University Medical Center
Omaha, Nebraska, USA
jwelie@creighton.edu

Robin Y. Wood, EdD, RN
Associate Professor and Coordinator of Learning Resource Centers
Connell School of Nursing
Boston College
Chestnut Hill, Massachusetts, USA
woodr@mail.bc.edu

Marylou Yam, PhD, RN
Associate Dean of Nursing
St. Peter's College
Jersey City, NJ, USA
myam@spc.edu

22. Index

1971 World Synod of Catholic Bishops, 51, 71
32nd General Congregation, 10, 50, 52-54, 56, 58, 62, 64, 65, 85, 116
33rd General Congregation, 54
34th General Congregation, 10, 53, 63

Academic freedom, 25, 27
Access to health care, 111, 127, 131, 170
  role of care givers, 112, 114
Achaerandio, 86
Action as hallmark of Jesuit education, 38
Admissions policies, 63, 127, 140-142, 150, 239
Affirmative action, 143
Agency for Health Care Policy and Research, 222
AIDS, 62, 98, 100-101, 176-180, 183, 203-209
Alcala, 33
Altruism, 119, 133-135, 146, 148
Alumni, *see* Students-Alumni
Alzheimer's dementia, 125
American Association of Colleges of Nursing, 211, 216
American Cancer Society, 194, 199
American College of Dentists, 115, 129, 185
American College of Obstetricians and Gynecologists, 199
American Dental Association, 114
American Medical Association, 140
American State Department, 54
Anatomy, 231-232
Annas, 195, 199
Appleyard, 23-26, 35, 44
Aquaviva, 34
Arrupe, 9-11, 15, 35, 51-52, 55-56, 66, 84, 85, 91
Association of Episcopal Colleges, 20, 42, 44
Ateneo de Zamboanga, 227
Attitude, *see* Motivation
Ayers, 185-191

Baer, 219, 222
Bandura, 195, 199, 213-214, 216
Barden, 194, 197, 200
Barnds, 22, 44
Basic health care, 120, 124, 158, 159
Bauer, 213, 218
Beck, 216, 217
Becker, 215-217
Beech, 194, 197, 200
Beirne, 86-88, 90, 91
Beirut, 51
Belgium, 231-233
Bellah, 102, 106, 108
Benin, 232
Bernstein, 194, 197, 199
Bernt, 161-168
Bethea, 212, 217
Bevilacqua, 155, 157
Biomedical research, *see* Research
Bioethics education, 138, 163, 170
Blot, 194, 200
Bodden, 194, 200

Bognet, 155-160
Boston College, 10, 193, 203-205
Boyles, 151
Brann, 137, 150
Breast cancer, 99, 193-201
Brown, 195, 199
Buchanan, 148, 150
Buddha, 83
Burack, 194, 199
Burkhardt, 44, 95-109
Butts, 220, 222

Cahill, 97, 108
Callahan, 32, 33, 40, 44-45, 173
Cameron, 151
Campbell A, 162, 167
Campbell J, 212-213, 217
Canon Law, 27
Carbone, 151
Carlson, 217
Catholic Health Association, 100
Catholic Health World, 100-101, 108
Catholic higher education
  academic freedom, 25, 27
  administrators, 29
  and the Vatican, 26
  canon law, 27
  church governance, 27
  faculty, 29
  history, 23
  identity, 23, 25
  in the modern world, 26-28
  lay boards, 24, 25
  models, 23-25
Catholic Hospital Association, 89
Catholic Relief Services, 166
Catholic Relief Services, 164, 166
Catholic universities, *see* Catholic higher education

CELAM, 78
Centesimus Annus, 79
Centro Juan B. Montalvo, 166
Cepress, 100, 108
Cesareo, 23, 26, 44
Champion, 194, 200
Characteristics of Jesuit education, 35-39, 59
  conscientization, 10, 37, 133-134, 140, 150, 167, 172
  modern, 36-39, 59
  promotion of justice, 84
  The Characteristics of Jesuit Education, 35-37
  whole person, 59
Charity
  versus justice, 51, 70, 84, 117, 123, 145
Children, 98, 111, 125
Chisholm L, 42, 44
Chisholm M, 208
Chittister, 34, 44
Civil rights movement, 24, 99
Clark L, 208
Clark P, 161-168
Clarkson, Bishop Robert Harper Clarkson, 21
Clarkson College, 20-22, 41
Clement XIV, 9
Clinical care, 124
Codina, 34, 44
Cohen, 194, 200
Coker, 212, 217
Coleman, 31, 32, 44
Collins, 46, 47, 151, 218
Colombia, 54
Commitment, *see* Motivation
Conscientization, *see* Characteristics of Jesuit education
Congo, 232

Connell School of Nursing, 193, 203
Connelly, 145, 150-151
Context as hallmark of Jesuit education, 37
Cope, 151, 213, 214
Costanza, 195, 199
Courses, *see* Curriculum; Subjects to be taught
Crandall, 146, 150
Creighton University, 12, 22, 40-43, 117, 128, 166, 176, 178, 181, 185-188
Cristobal, 227-230
Crowley, 23, 35, 45
Cuellar, 220, 222
Cultural competence, 171; *see also* Prejudice
Cuomo, 97, 102, 108
Cura personalis, 161, 235, 239; *see also* Whole person
Curriculum, 124-127, 149, 161-164, 175-178, 180-183, 229, 231-234 *See also* Subjects to be taught

Dabney, 222
Daoust, 10, 15
Davis KJ, 194, 200
Davis FD, 235-240
Day, 32, 45
Debt, *see* tuition
DeJong, 198-199
DeMarco, 203-209
Demoustier, 84, 91
Dental hygiene, 12, 112-114
Dentistry, 12, 111-130, 155, 177, 185-191
Diakonia fidei, *see* Service of faith
Dinemann, 217

Disabilities, 106, 112, 126, 177, 181, 197, 198, 219, 232
Discrimination in health care, *see* Health disparities; Poor-marginalized medically
Distribution of wealth, 58, 71, 81, 86
in health care, 111
Doctor-patient relationship, *see* Therapeutical relationship
Doctors Without Borders, 167, 177
Dominican Republic, 164, 186, 189
Dorr, 90, 91
Dorsey, 222
Downey, 31, 45
Duffy, 195, 201
Duminuco, 35-37, 45, 47
Dunn, 218
Dutton, 213, 217

Eagleson, 78, 91, 92
Economic justice for all, 81
Education, *see* Health sciences education
Edwards, 194, 200
El Salvador, 87
Elderly, 99, 107, 125, 194
Ellacuría, 56, 64, 66, 86, 88-91
Ellard, 141, 150
Ellis, 45
Emblen, 45
Emergency medical services, 12
Episcopalian Church, 20
Esthetic surgery and dentistry, 126
Ethical erosion, *see* Health sciences education-dehumanization
Ethics, *see* Bioethics
Ethics education, *see* Bioethics education

Evaluation as hallmark of Jesuit education, 39, 239
Ex Corde Ecclesiae, 27-29, 65
Experience as hallmark of Jesuit education, 38
Experiential learning, see Service learning
Externships, 166, 169, 171, 180; see also Service learning; Service trips

Facultés Universitaires Notre-Dame de la Paix, 231-233
Faculty, see Jesuit universities-faculty; Role models
Faith versus science, 12, 26-29, 40, 61, 63
Farmer, 159, 160
Faulkner, 144, 150
Feeling, its role in education, 38
Feeney, 29, 45
Film, 181, 203, 205, 208
Finding God in all things, 32
Fineberg, 209
Flaskerud, 212, 217
Fleming, 212, 218
Fordham University, 128
Formation, 59
France, 9
Freeman, 194-195, 199, 216
Freire, 165
Friedman, 194, 197, 199

Gable, 209
Gamm, 219, 221, 222
Ganss, 122, 129
Gaudium et Spes, 70, 77
Gedeit, 148, 150
General Congregation of the Society of Jesus, 55, 58, 61, 65, 66; *see also* numbers (e.g, 32nd GC)

George, 99, 194, 199
Georgetown University, 40, 45, 95, 102, 105, 108, 128, 182, 235-240
Gibbon, 151
Gielen, 217
Gilman, 29, 45
Ginzberg, 137, 150
Glaser, 151
God's Lost Children, 98
Gold, 194, 200
Goldberg, 218
Gorman, 108
Graef, 134-135, 150
Graves, 34, 45
Gray, 23-26, 35, 44
Greater glory of God, 65
Griffin, 131, 150
Gurney, 104, 194, 199
Gutierrez, 91

Haiti, 156-160, 166
Hall, 199, 215, 217
Hanusa, 151
Harney, 128-129
Harras, 194, 200
Harvanek, 34, 45
Harvard University, 102
Harvey, 151
Health, 169
  as social good, 97
  as wholeness, 102
Health administration, 12
Health as liberation, 162
Health care
  access, 111
  and promotion of justice, 106
  as profession, 114
  financing, 135
  Jesuit involvement in, 123

Index

Health Care Financing Administration, 197, 200
Health disparities, 111, 114, 194
  research, 195
  research funding, 121
Health sciences education, 236
  dehumanization, 119, 134-139, 145, 235-239
  externship, 180
  financing, 119, 135
  see also Curriculum
Heft, 23-25, 27, 28, 45
Helping and Healing, 14, 127, 184
Higher education
  student expectations, 102
Higher Education Committee, 59
Hilfiker, 139, 140, 150, 178
Hippocratic tradition, 134
Hiring, 64
Hiroshima, 9
HIV, *see* AIDS
Hogar Luby, 166
Holy Cross College, 45
Homelessness, 98
Hôpital Lumière in Bonne Fin (Haiti), 156
Horizon of concern, 88
Hrubetz, 117, 129
Human Development Report, 58
Humanism, 34, 143
  in health care, 104, 133
  see also Health sciences education-dehumanization
Hutchison, 222
Hyland, 156

Ignatian Pedagogy: A Practical Approach, 37
Ignatius, 9, 13, 19, 30-34, 37, 38, 42-44, 47, 54, 57, 66, 83, 84, 121-123, 129, 169, 173
  own education, 33
ILAC, *see* Institute of Latin American Concern
Ilness
  and injustice, 97
  and social conditions, 97, 102, 140, 170
  and violence, 98
  chronic, 125
  terminal, 125
Immigrants, 50, 57
Indian Health Service, 177
Individualism, 101
  and promotion of justice, 106
Injustice
  and illness, 97
  distribution of wealth, 58, 71, 81, 86
Inquisition, 32
Institute of Latin American Concern, 166, 178, 185-191
International Center for Jesuit Education, 45
International Commission on the Apostolate of Jesuit Education, 35
Inui, 143, 144, 150

Jacobs, 218
Jain, 148, 150
Jesuit education
  and promotion of justice, 56
  documents, *see Ratio Studiorum; Characteristics of Jesuit Education; Ignatian Pedagogy*
  early characteristics, 34
  identity, 34

International Commission on the Apostolate of Jesuit Education, 35
investment, 55
professions, 61
versus social apostolate, 52
See also Characteristics of Jesuit Education; Ratio Studiorum
Jesuit Educational Quarterly, 13
Jesuit health sciences education
  school founding, 227-230
  early history, 122
  financing, 119, 121
  first medical school, 122
  identity, 117-119
  missions, 144
  number of university programs, 12, 122
  school closings, 122
  see also Jesuit universities
Jesuit pedagogy, *see* Jesuit education
Jesuit Refugee Service, 62, 166
Jesuit Secondary Education Association, 56, 66
Jesuit universities
  and promotion of justice, 116, 117
  faculty, 29, 43, 62, 239
  first school, 30
  health sciences, 117-120
  history, 30
  identity, 59, 63, 64
  missions, 59, 123
  original purpose, 12
  partnerships, 62-63
  promotion of justice, 86
  research mission, 61
  status as university, 11, 35, 63-64
  suppression, 31, 122
  see also Jesuit health sciences education
John Paul II, 23, 27, 29, 47, 60-67, 78-80, 92
John XXIII, 77, 91
Johnson C, 208
Johnson E, 23, 45
Jones, 23, 25, 45, 217
Jonsen, 133, 134, 150
Justice
  as fidelity, 103
  as love, 103
  as social contract, 145
  cultural determinants, 81
  in the Bible, 103
  theories, 14, 72, 128, 134, 144
  versus charity, 51, 70, 84, 117, 123, 145
  see also Social contract

Kane, 194, 200
Kaplan, 209
Kay, 146, 150
Kerner, 194, 195, 199
King, 30, 122, 212, 217
Kissell, 9-13, 175-184
Kolvenbach, 11, 13, 19, 23, 30, 32, 35-39, 43-46, 49-67, 85, 91, 116, 122-123, 129, 166, 171, 173, 211, 214, 217
Koop, 162, 167
Kopelman, 145, 150
Kosary, 194, 200
Ku, 194, 200
Kub, 217

Land O'Lakes conference, 25
Lannin, 194, 200
Lannon, 29, 46
Larson, 46

Latin America, 51, 81-82, 85
Lauver, 194, 200
Law, 70, 117
  exclusion from Jesuit universities, 13, 122
Lay boards, 24
Lempert, 213, 217
Leo XIII, 77
Liban, 232
Liberation, 78, 79
  1971 World Synod of Catholic Bishops, 51
  pedagogy, 165
  theology, 80, 165
Linn, 143, 151
Loemker, 150
Lonergan, 157
Loyola (Spain), 83
Loyola Institute, 47
Loyola University Chicago, 128
Loyola University Stritch School of Medicine, 14
Ludmerer, 135, 142, 145, 147, 149, 151
Lynch G, 157
Lynch M, 208
Lyons, 164

Madagascar, 232
Madan, 194, 197, 200
Maddux, 218
Maher, 30, 33-35, 46
Maibach, 213, 217
Mandelblatt, 194, 200
Managed care, see Access; Health care-financing; Health sciences education-financing
Marginalization in health care, see Health disparities; Poor-marginalized medically

Markkula Center for Applied Ethics, 169-173
Marquette University, 128
Marshburn, 198, 200
Martín-Baró, 86
Marxism, 54
Massaro 69-92
Matthews H, 194, 200
Matthews R, 33, 34, 46
Mauksch, 145, 151
Maxwell, 168
McBrien, 32, 46
McCullough, 46
McCurdy, 144, 150
McGeady, 108-109
McGrath, 96, 108
McKeown, 212, 217
McMurtrie, 23, 35, 46
Medellin, 81, 116
Medical education, see Health sciences education
Medical ethics education, see Bioethics education
Medical missions, 156, 230; see also Institute for Latin American Concern
Medicine, 70, 95, 103-107, 111-130, 131-151, 157-161, 169-171, 176, 181, 227-240
  art and science, 132
  commercialization, 133
  curriculum, 126
  exclusion from Jesuit universities, 13, 122
  Jesuit involvement in, 103
  limits thereof, 170
Men and women for others, 10, 12, 36, 56, 116, 167
Menon, 194, 200
Mercondante, 218

Messina, 30, 84
Mexico, 79
Middleman, 215, 218
Miles, 138, 139, 151
Miller B, 194, 200
Miller K, 208
Minorities, 99, 171, 194
   minority students, 127
Mitchell, 194, 200
Modras, 30, 46
Modus Parisiensis, 33
Montserrat, 32
Morris, 195, 201
Morrison, 30, 46
Moser, 28, 46
Moses, 98, 99, 194, 200
Motivation, 26, 38-39, 75, 125-128, 133-139, 143-149, 157, 189, 219, 239
Murder of UCA Jesuits, 88
Murkowski, 148, 150
Murphy, 213, 217
Muth, 194, 195, 199
Mutschler, 194, 197, 199

National Conference of Catholic Bishops, 46
National Health Service Corps, 137
National Institutes of Health, 129, 195, 200
National Institute of Dental and Craniofacial Research, 112, 128, 129
National Rural Health Association, 219, 223
Native Americans, 21, 22, 42, 101, 177
   Ponca, 22
   Sioux, 22
Neff, 194, 197, 199
Nelson, 140, 151

Networking, 232
Newland, 140, 151
NIH, *see* National Institutes of Health
Nobili, 49
Norris, 203-209
Notre Dame, 24
Notre Dame University, 23
Nurse practitioners, 219
Nursing, 117, 118, 177, 190, 203, 205, 206, 209, 222
   research, 193-201, 211-218, 219-223
Nursing home, 99, 125, 126, 148, 177

Occupational therapy, 12
Oh, 215, 217
Optometry, 148
Oral Health Care in America, 112
Ouzts, 140, 151
O'Brien D, 23, 25, 35, 46
O'Brien DJ, 67, 92
O'Campo, 217
O'Connor Hospital Board of Directors, 170-173
O'Hare, 46
O'Malley A, 194, 200
O'Malley J, 30-31, 35, 46
O'Toole, 147, 151

Padberg, 32, 43, 47, 95
Paris, University of, 33
Parker J, 29, 45
Parker K, 30, 33, 35, 46
Parker S, 194, 200
Passon, 29, 47
Pasternak, 155, 160
Pastoral care, *see* Service of faith

Patient
  as a person, 104
  as God's image, 107
  vulnerability, 124
  whole person, 104
Paul VI, 71, 77-78, 81, 92
Pearson, 167
Peck, 20-47
Pedagogy, *see* Jesuit education
Pellegrino, 9, 14, 15, 117, 127-129, 184
Personalist ethics, 104, 107
Petrie, 146, 151
Pharmacy, 12, 118, 177, 187, 190
Philippines, 227-230
Phillips J, 194
Phillips R, 209
Physical therapy, 12, 20, 125, 180
Piront, 231-233
Pius VII, 9
Plan to Eliminate Health Disparities, 112
Platt D, 33, 34, 46
Platt M, 157
Plichta, 212, 218
Pont-à-Mousson (France), 122
Poor/poverty 157
  and illness, 112
  categories, 97
  cries of the poor, 97-101
  in medical education and research, 62, 119, 215
  in the Bible, 97
  marginalized medically, 124-25, 176, 194, 213, 228
  minorities, 176
  seeing the world through their eyes, 62, 70, 82, 88, 103, 149, 162, 164, 171, 181, 191
  stigmatizing medical conditions, 126, 176
  in the Scriptures, 72-76
Populorum Progressio, 78
Poverty, *see* Poor
Preferential option for the poor
  alternate phrasings, 79
  and education, 84
  as conflict, 80, 82, 87
  as epistemology, 70
  first use, 71
  grounded in faith, 79
  Ignatian roots, 83
  in education, 61
  precursors, 77
  translation to health care, 89
  versus charity, 117
  versus Marxism, 80
  versus social Darwinism, 76
Pregus, 218
Prejudice, 136, 143, 148, 157, 162, 164, 171; *see also* Cultural competence
Premedical education, 140-142, 156, 161
  service trips, 156
  See also Undergraduate education
Prentice, 199, 217, 218
Primary care, 124, 126, 136, 145, 159, 198
Privilege, 96
Profession, 114
Professional education, 61, 117, 120, 134, 139, 144, 176
  promotion of justice, 123
Promotion of justice, 54, 65
  and education, 56
  and service of faith, 10, 11, 44, 50, 52, 54-56, 63, 65, 79, 231
  early criticism, 52

preparatory education, 123-126, 156, 161, 171, 178, 189, 211
service trips, 54
versus Marxism, 54
Public health, 97, 113, 162, 163, 228-230
Puebla, 71, 78-81
Puebla Final Document, 71, 92
Puhl, 47
Purtilo, 175

Quiroga, 213, 218

Racism, *see* Prejudice
Ratio Studiorum, 33, 34; *see also* Jesuit education
Rawl, 194, 200
Reflection as hallmark of Jesuit education, 38
Refusal to provide care, 131, 138, 139
Register, 218
Reid, 198, 200
Relationship between care giver and patient, *see* Therapeutical relationship
Rerum Novarum, 77
Research, 61, 111-130, 136, 232; *see also* Nursing-research
Residency training, 134, 135
Ries, 194, 200, 201
Robbins, 151
Robert Wood Johnson Foundation, 121
Rodriguez, 213, 218
Role models, 136-138, 147, 148, 239
Roman College, 31, 34
Rosenberg, 194, 201
Ruanda, 232
Ruiz, 209
Rural health care, 137, 143, 166, 177, 180-181, 185, 187, 191, 219-223, 227-230

Saint Francis of Assisi, 83
Saint Joseph's University, 161, 164
Saint Louis University, 23, 24, 117, 128
Saint Peter's College, 214
San Salvador, 85, 87
Sanders, 168
Sanford, 219-223
Santa Clara University, 10-12, 49, 56, 66, 90, 116-117, 122, 169-173, 193, 199, 203, 205
Sawyers, 46
Scharper, 91, 92
Schlegel, 41, 47
Schoelenberger, 217
Schulman, 169-173
Schwarz, 167
Scroope, 32, 45
Self-interest, *see* Altruism
Sen, 82, 92
Service, 203, 205
Service learning, 60, 63, 118, 126, 137, 147-148, 156-159, 166, 185, 187, 189, 191, 239
care for persons, 106
Service of faith, 12, 19, 30, 52-54, 56, 63
versus social apostolate, 79
see also Promotion of justice-and service of faith
Sharkey, 32, 37, 38, 47
Sherer, 215, 218
Shinagawa, 194, 200
Shore, 30, 33-35, 46
Siddharthan, 198, 200

Siegel, 105, 108, 109
Sifri, 148, 151
Skupinki, 213, 218
Smith L, 219, 222
Smith P, 212, 217
Sobrino, 86, 88, 90, 91
Social accountability budgets, 89
Social contract, 103, 144
Social Darwinism
  versus preferential option for the poor, 76
Society of Jesus
  Constitutions, 34
  Higher Education Committee, 59
  history, 83
  investment in education, 55
  involvement in health care, 103-104, 123
  missions, 9, 52
  modern history, 84
  reestablishment, 9
  suppression, 9, 31
Soeken, 212-213, 217
solidarity, 60, 78, 159
Sollicitudo Rei Socialis, 79
Spain, 9
Spiritual Exercises, 30, 31
  impact on education, 33
  origins, 32
  purpose, 32
Spirituality
  Ignatian, 32
  role in education, 41
  versus religion, 31
Spring Hill College, 219, 222
Steinbach, 148, 151
Stempsey, 131-151
Stoto, 209

Students
  alumni, 155
  attitudes, 135
  educational debt, *see* Tuition
  expectations, 102
Stuifbergen, 215, 217
Subjects to be taught, 124, 126
  art, 30
  drama, 30
  ethics, 232
  Greek, 34
  languages, 34, 157, 166, 188, 189, 198
  law, 13, 122
  literature and medicine, 161
  medicine, 13, 122
  music, 30
  opera, 30
  philosophy, 232
  psychology, 232
  religious sciences, 232
  rhetoric, 34
  theology and medicine, 161
  See also Curriculum
Swartzberg, 151
Switzer, 151

Taylor, 148, 151
Theories of Justice, *see* Justice-theories
Therapeutical relationship, 104, 140, 158
  and promotion of justice, 103, 104
Thomasma, 2, 9, 14, 15, 117, 127-129, 184
Thuman, 168
Tisdell, 31, 47
Toton, 167, 168
Townsend-Rocchiccioli, 222, 223

Trickle-down economics, 81
Trussell, 209
Tuition, 86, 119, 121, 137
Tylenda, 47
Tyson, 212, 218

UCA, 85-87
  murder of Jesuits, 88
Undergraduate education, 156, 161, 169
  externship, 169-172
  service trips, 166
  see also Premedical education
United Nations Development Program, 58, 75
United States Catholic Bishops, 82, 92
United States Department of Agriculture Economic Research Servic, 219
United States Public Health Service, 112
Universidad Centroamericana José Simeón Cañas, see UCA
Université Saint-Joseph (Beirut), 51, 123
Universities
  Catholic, see Catholic higher education
  Medieval history, 33
University of Detroit-Mercy, 10, 128
University of Nebraska Medical Center, 181, 183, 228-232, 235-238, 240
University of Paris, 33, 34
University of Scranton, 156
  Medical Alumni Council, 155

Valencia (Spain), 10

Vanderford, 194, 200
Vatican Congregation for the Doctrine of the Faith, 80
Vatican Council II, 24-25, 50, 70, 77
Veysey, 23, 47
Vietnam, 232
Vietnam War, 24
Viseltear, 136, 137, 142, 151
Vocation, 14, 19, 43, 61, 128, 171, 184
Volk, 150
Vulnerability, 127, 212
  and dependence, 99, 101
  and illness, 104, 139, 144
  children, 98
  dependence, 99
  elderly, 99
  minorities, 99
  patients, 124
  see also Poor
Walsh, 32, 47
Watson, 138, 151
Way of proceeding, 63, 84
Webb, 194, 197, 199
Welie, 9-13, 111-130, 212, 215
Werner, 162, 165, 168
Weston, 168
White G, 151
White K, 145, 151
Whole person, 59-61, 104, 117, 161, 235
William F. Connell School of Nursing, see Connell School of Nursing
Wilson, 27, 28, 47
Wingo, 194, 200, 201
Witt, 151
Wood G, 215, 218
Wood R, 193-201

World Health Organization, 111, 129, 228
World Synod of Catholic Bishops, 51, 54, 67, 71, 92
Wynne, 217

Yale University, 135
Yam, 211-218

Zamboanga Medical School Foundation, 227-230